Saving the Heart of American Health Care

Saving the Heart of American Health Care

How Patients and Their Doctors Can Mend a Broken System

KENNETH P. ANDERSON D.O., MS, CPE

ISBN-13: 9781983745850
ISBN-10: 1983745855
Library of Congress Control Number: 2018900689
CreateSpace Independent Publishing Platform
North Charleston, South Carolina

*To my parents, Ted and Kay Anderson, and my brother, Mike—who taught me
the values of hard work, determination, and curiosity
To my wife, Dyan—who stands beside me daily in the pursuit of my dreams
To Jennifer, Andy, Cassie, Eric, Zach, Elyse, Alex, Elsie, Leif, Pat, and Brendan,
with the hope that they will find a kind and caring health-care system that ful-
fills their needs to achieve great health, long life, and
glorious well-being
To my mentors, Dr. Jeremy Swan, Dr. Abraham Tobas, Dr. Bruno Masters,
and Phil Newbold, who encouraged me to set my sights on the stars but to keep
my feet on the ground
To all of my patients and coworkers who showed me how to care with caring and
to conspire with them around the values of strength, honesty,
and courage*

Contents

Section 3
The Path Forward

Section 1
The Historical Context

INTRODUCTION TO SECTION 1
THE SOCIAL COMPACT FOR AMERICAN HEALTH CARE

No longer do Americans enjoy the best health-care delivery system in the world. As costs continue their unrelenting spiral upward and as clinical outcomes lag behind the rest of the industrialized world, those who deliver health care and those who receive that care are left with a melancholy realization that much has changed, and not all for the better. American health-care technology continues its scientific advance, but the care experience has deteriorated to become an often unsatisfying and unrecognizable transaction. Although many would describe the disorganized and complex American health-care delivery system as itself being on life support, both care consumers and providers remain hopeful that the magic of a meaningful and human care experience can be recovered and held to its appropriate place of high regard. Separated only by the narrow distance of a stethoscope, what can health-care participants do to demand that no health-care delivery system should be built without our joint involvement and leadership? To better arm ourselves for this political combat, we first need to explore the winding path that resulted in our being at this exact moment in health-care history.

As a naïve high-school foreign-exchange student to Costa Rica in 1969, I was presented with my first lessons regarding the many layers of opportunity that are found across multiple strata of "persons of privilege." While I was attending classes in the rural town of Grecia, known best for its lush mountain-grown coffee fields, my adoptive uncle became sick with a cough and fever. As I arrived home after school, I wondered why someone wouldn't just put him in a car or call an ambulance so that he could seek the advice of the nearest local physician. Over several days, my uncle's health continued to decline, and without antibiotics and a hospital bed with oxygen and pulmonary therapy, he passed into unconsciousness and died.

Reflecting on those very scary days, I was at first confused and angry about the unjust situation that had befallen a man with whom I had shared a tight family bond during Saturday-evening extended-family fiestas and Sunday soccer games after Catholic mass. The dichotomy of health-care services available to me as an American versus what was available to my Costa Rican uncle was made even more evident by the contrast between my uncle's struggle with pneumonia and the great celebration of technology witnessed worldwide with the first lunar landing, described as "one small step for man, one giant leap for mankind." My overwhelming uneasiness and anger were gradually replaced by an emerging adolescent idealism, and I vowed to take up the banner of health-care delivery so that I could return one day to my adopted land to help others like my uncle. As a good student of science and math, I was soon able to transform my passion for basic scientific fact-finding into interest in a career where I could use this raw knowledge to help my community—my personal mission was set. All that I needed to do was to spend the next fifteen years perfecting my craft, and I could then realize a deeply seated calling to return to Costa Rica to help those most in need of health-care services. Although yet to occur, the personal mission launched by my time there continues to drive my quest to help make health-care experiences better.

During my educational experiences, I met and learned from some of the best minds in health care, directly acquiring the medical knowledge needed to engage in the health-care dance with my patients. Of equal importance, I learned from a few mentors the awkward lessons related to how *not* to deliver care, observing the style of a few who appeared to be less than fully committed to participating in an intensely human health-care delivery experience. I was never able to reconcile the apparent incivility of those few who appeared detached from the human side of this very personal transaction. From the immense sense of duty and privilege I felt during my fleeting interactions with patients and their families, I remained in awe of the courage that I witnessed each day as vulnerable people wrestled with their own life-and-death struggles while battling cancer, stroke, and other chronic illnesses. In addition to the medical and surgical expertise required to wage war against disease, these brave warriors appeared to be looking for a gentle heart and a listening ear of a clinician who could reach across the stethoscope to complete the unique bond that was called the "physician-patient relationship." This, I was later to surmise, is what lies at the very core of the professional role of a care provider. The experience of authentically caring for and about another person in need is more than just a business proposition with a narrow focus of translating patient needs into meeting one's own selfish financial goals.

Throughout my forty years as a medical student, intern, resident, subspecialist health-care provider, administrator, policy maker, and mentor to physicians in training, my quest has always been to keep the human side of care delivery front and center, reminding each of my colleagues to focus on an image of a physician delivering care to their mother or father, or even more personally, how they would feel when presented with their own health-care challenges. When young practitioners allowed themselves the ability to personalize this applied science, they could then embrace the beauty of the care experience and relish a newfound sense of privilege of providing care for others that would yield the greatest intrinsic reward from their profession.

This book is intended for both the health-care provider and the health-care consumer, to better understand the personal impact resulting from the changes introduced in health-care delivery that I witnessed over the arc of my career. In his work *The Social Transformation of American Medicine*, Dr. Paul Starr underscores the political and societal issues that have been in play for over a century that shaped the American health-care system into its current form. Missing from this discussion, however, is the personal impact on the social compact that had been built between providers and consumers that made health care the most human of all experiences, providing immense personal reward for health-care practitioners and their patients. By exploring the human emotions associated with these changing policy proposals, I will use the knowledge gained from the multiple perspectives of my nearly forty years of health-care experience to assist those who are responsible for creating further changes in the oversight and financing of care delivery systems. If the proposed changes incorporate these lessons learned from providing care with caring, we will as a nation be able to continue our path toward delivering health outcomes that outpace the rest of the world, and we will avoid the negative consequences that might be expected from these restructuring activities.

One

CONNECTING TO THE HEART OF HEALTH CARE

For more than two centuries, the ritual of senior physicians "making rounds" with younger doctors in training has provided an educational experience leading to the transfer of medical knowledge gained through years of observation, research, and clinical experience. Often taking the form of a small and meandering mob moving from patient room to patient room in a teaching hospital, these conversations serve as defining moments of truth for medical students and young physicians where each is prompted to orally deliver reports about patient progress or to recite medical literature verbatim as it relates to specific patient-care conundrums. One common theme emerging from these encounters is the direct and sometimes critical commentary of learned individuals hoping to pass on their wisdom, and the styles used to deliver this knowledge can be highly variable. Some senior doctors use a Socratic method of rapid-fire question-and-answer sessions designed to break down a young trainee and to remind junior physicians just how much more remains to be learned. Other mentor physicians choose to adopt a more academic approach using brief lectures on esoteric topics tied to that physician's research and clinical strengths.

The spectrum of possibilities from these teaching events makes them memorable for several reasons, and the lessons that arise from such gut-wrenching experiences burn long-lasting and deep holes into the emotional psyches of young and often immature trainees. As new medical careers are launched, these lessons travel with them, to be applied during times of high emotional stress such as when making life-and-death decisions, and some lessons are crafted as teaching points that remind the protégé that health care continues to be a very human endeavor. Some of these lasting stories are derived from experiences that young clinicians hopes never to repeat, such as a careless medication error or a botched surgical procedure, while more victorious experiences reinforce the beauty of the profession that chose them as guardians to whom the future of health-care delivery could be entrusted.

This memory-building exercise applies not only to the technical aspects of delivering care, but also to the ways in which senior clinicians model behaviors needed to provide care for their patients. Some of these lessons are reinforced because of the positive nature of the provider-patient bond, such as when a senior clinician stops to thoroughly answer questions posed by a patient's family or an exemplary practitioner holds the hand of a dying patient. Some experiences are best recalled as being "lessons in how *not* to practice medicine," as demonstrated by ego-swollen clinicians whose main job is to remind those in their midst just how lucky they are to have such a superdoctor as a mentor. To some educators, patients are just the annoying inconvenience of their craft, a necessary evil in the practice of medicine. Lessons learned in the presence of such physicians become the substrate for ever-growing tales of terror from one medical school class to the next.

During my early training experiences, my fellow residents and I frequently reminded one another that learning could come in all forms, one of which was in rejecting moments of impersonal communication. By doing so, we could perform better at a future time when we were personally accountable for delivering a more compassionate care experience. One such example of a clinician with little time for patients and trainees was a transplant physician who was stopped by another senior attending doctor to inquire how the clinical work-up of a prospective organ donor was progressing. The transplant physician, never known for his caring attitude, turned to his assistant and muttered, "Don't these people know how busy I am? Please ask them to make an appointment if they want to discuss patient care with us." Although this was an atypical teaching moment for impressionable young doctors in training, it remains one that stands out as I think back to the many other notable examples of human interaction modeled by other highly respected physicians who happened to have mastered the medical art that care and caring should not be separated.

Sitting at the end of a long and spotless walnut table surrounded by sixteen chairs, Dr. H. J. C. "Jeremy" Swan was beginning another of his weekly "brandy rounds" designed to download the many teaching lessons that had occurred that week at Cedars-Sinai Medical Center in Los Angeles. A standing-room-only crowd filled the room, and squeezed around the table were more residents, cardiology fellows, and medical students than could be comfortably seated, each hanging on to every word uttered by one of the true "gentlemen of medicine." Dr. Swan, a peaceful and small man with silver-white hair, had been called to sunny Los Angeles from the Mayo Clinic in Rochester, Minnesota, years earlier to help stimulate clinical and basic research on cardiovascular disease. He and his longtime friend and research associate, Dr. William "Willie" Ganz, used the simple observation of watching the sails of boats launched from the Santa Monica harbor to design a diagnostic device that bore their names. With their sails unfurled so as to catch the wind, these sailboats inspired the two scientists to innovate a design that allowed a vascular catheter to be propelled using the body's natural circulation to arrive at a spot where measurements of distant heart chamber pressures could be taken from inside a blood vessel. The Swan-Ganz catheter had become a mainstay in intensive care units across the country by the time I arrived as a visiting family-medicine resident from Iowa, and I wanted to hear firsthand about how this technology had allowed for miracles to occur in managing patients with heart attacks. In these patients, knowledge about the delicate balance of fluids filling the heart was needed to precisely adjust medications to hold even a glimmer of hope for recovery.

As five o'clock drew near, the first of many small brandy glasses was being prepared and offered by the Irish sage as he launched a discussion on the "clinical pearls" of the week. I was just one year removed from medical school, and lessons like these left me awestruck as I gained the firsthand experience I would need to help my future patients. Sipping slowly, Dr. Swan neatly replaced his small snifter glass back on the long, dark wood table and pulled a stethoscope from the pocket of his tweed jacket. "Does anyone in this room know what this is?" he asked quite innocently. We looked around the convocation as if asking one another whether someone had hijacked Dr. Swan's body and removed all the knowledge that had at one time flowed through its veins. Finally, a first-year cardiology fellow sarcastically chimed in, "It's called a stethoscope!"

Slowly drawing in another sip of brandy, Dr. Swan softly replied, "Of course it is. Don't any of you ever forget what this little device is used for and that you should never replace the most effective clinical instrument ever created with cold and impersonal technology alone." As he began to describe the tried-and-true methods of physical diagnosis and compassionate historical questioning that had launched his career in Ireland so many years previously, the world of clinical cardiology came alive, and the greatest lessons that came from these Friday brandy rounds were more about the art of taking care of a patient in need rather than about the filling pressures found inside the heart's chambers. This "old man of cardiology" gave each of us a powerful reminder that the practice of medicine is foremost about being human, and since compassion lay at the very heart of this very human practice, we were all charged to uphold a lifelong commitment to caring for and about others in need of our expertise.

Some years before the encounter with Dr. Swan, as I was just beginning my medical school education, I had been assigned to a clinical rotation in the busy emergency department of a local teaching hospital, learning about the proper application of orthopedic splints and casts, management of fluid overload in patients with kidney failure, and the stepwise protocols to respond to a patient whose heart had suddenly stopped. While intently involved in learning from the physicians who were only too willing to challenge my knowledge deficits, I happened across a nephrology fellow who was moonlighting in the emergency room to earn a few extra dollars by picking up an additional shift. Like a puppy in search of approval from its owner, I asked every question I could of this brilliant young physician who was nearing the end of her formal medical training journey. Dr. Linda Francisco seemed to possess an immense amount of practical knowledge about all matters medical, and during a break between patients, I asked her about how her interest in health-care delivery had begun. By reflecting on her own journey into health-care delivery, the senior trainee was able to paint a vivid picture of what I was to experience in my pursuit of a personal calling to deliver medical care.

Dr. Francisco said that as the daughter of a small-town family physician, she had little choice but to select a career in health since she possessed talents in applied science, and she received a healthy nudge from her father as they discussed her prospective career choices. Of the five children born to Dr. Sidney Frederick Yugend and his wife, Harriet Bertine Hooper, three had developed an interest in health care, but only one had chosen to follow the patriarch into the direct practice of medicine. Embracing the life of a small-town general practitioner, Dr. Yugend wore several hats in caring for his community, taking on the roles of surgeon, obstetrician, pediatrician, and family physician. He had arrived in Des Moines, Iowa, following his graduation from the University of Minnesota in 1939 to launch a medical career in a small town just south of the capital city that would span his entire working life. In fact, just a few weeks following the completion of a one-year internship in Des Moines, Sidney and Bertine were married, and when a patient of his went into labor on the day they exchanged their vows, the newlyweds drove to the hospital after the ceremony so that Sid could attend the birth of another new citizen of Indianola, Iowa. The following morning, without breaking stride and in the absence of a honeymoon, Dr. Yugend reported dutifully to his office, where a full slate of patients waited for him.

There were certainly some blurred lines between vocation and avocation for him, and the intense commitment he had made to his community of patients was not lost on his wife and children. Although he was a loving father who wanted to make certain that his family had the best things in life, Dr. Yugend never accompanied his loved ones on any of their carefully planned vacation trips. In fact, his work ethic demanded that he make himself available for his patients 24 hours a day, 7 days a week, and 365 days a year, taking no time off for relaxation. Even though his family understood the seriousness of his work and his commitment to an honored profession, the intense work schedule did take a toll on the relationship between husband and wife, leaving a sense of longing that was felt by family members who wanted him present to share their important bonding experiences. Dr. Yugend's belief was that since he had committed himself to his craft following medical school, he would find it extremely difficult to break away from his practice no matter how much his family wished he could.

As his medical practice continued into his later years, Dr. Yugend also served as the personal caregiver for his beloved wife, who was suffering the ravages of the late stages of Alzheimer's disease. As he was repositioning her in bed one afternoon, he suffered an acute bout of chest pain, for which he ultimately required emergency coronary artery bypass surgery. He spent the next week recuperating from surgery at the very hospital where he had admitted many of his own patients, a place where he had spent so many hours relieving the pain and suffering of others under his care. While he was recovering in the hospital, Dr. Yugend's wife passed away, and he came home to a very quiet and empty house. Trying to ready himself to return to practice, the only life he had ever known, he suddenly slumped over his desk at work and died, completing a life of medical practice that lasted right up until the moment when he took his last breath. Sidney and his wife died approximate three weeks apart, leaving four daughters and a lifetime of memories for his community.

In the big picture, the impact he left behind from a lifelong commitment to his medical practice was felt by a deeply devoted community, which continued to reach out to his children for years after his death to express gratitude for all that he had given. Dr. Francisco, now retired from a successful practice of medicine herself, later relayed that even if Dr. Yugend had wanted to reduce his workload, it would have been impossible, given the nature of the commitment he had made to his vocation and to the community. When asked if she had learned any lessons from watching her father deliver such committed care to his community, Dr. Francisco mentioned that she had made a pact with her husband, also a medical doctor, that they would try to deliver the very human care that had so well defined her father, but they would do so with greater work-life balance for the benefit of their own family.

As to the nature of the social compact that had been formed seventy-five years earlier between Dr. Yugend and his community, his daughter reflected that this "gentleman of medicine" would have "rolled over in his grave" if he could see how the practice of medicine is being performed today, where the strong presence of a physician in the community is but a fleeting memory and patients experience long delays as they attempt to access physicians to evaluate their medical problems. Although none of their children went into the practice of medicine, Dr. Francisco and her husband did continue the long tradition of family service to health care by supporting a daughter who became a dentist, in part because of the example provided by her parents' ability to set limits on the amount of time taken away from family activities.

Stories such as these are found throughout every community, hospital, and medical office in America, but the intense personal commitment to care and caring does appear to be waning in response to the many changes created by health-care policies that affect governance, oversight, and reimbursement of health care. For future generations of practitioners and patients to be able to experience the beauty of such human experiences created during the intense stress of illness and injury, the health-care delivery system will need to accommodate changes that maintain the human bond between those in need of care and those delivering it. If allowed to deteriorate into a series of cold and technical transactions, personal health-care experiences will be but a dream of past generations, leaving medical care in the hands of those wishing to design health care as a commodity. It's not too late to save the heart of health care, but it will take concerted effort by all parties in this great dance of life.

Two

Constructing Today's Health-Care Delivery System

No issue has created more public rancor in the past half century than the debate surrounding the best way to finance and provide access to health care for 325 million Americans. The resultant changes from health-care policies affecting cost, quality, and access to care have strained the intimate bond between care providers and care consumers to a breaking point. On January 21, 2017, just one day following the inauguration of Donald J. Trump as the forty-fifth president of the United States, over three million marchers gathered across the fifty states in part to protest the president's proposal to revoke a grand experiment in expanded access for health-care coverage.

The repeal of the Patient Protection and Affordable Care Act (ACA) was a core campaign promise of the incoming president with the full support of a Republican majority in both the House and the Senate. This new leadership coalition, swept into power by the very group of Americans who would most likely lose their existing benefits from the unwinding of the ACA, had been designing a proposal to repeal and replace "Obamacare" for nearly a decade. Lost in the national discussion of how health-care services might be assured at a price that would slow the escalating percentage of the nation's gross national product spent on health-care service delivery is the changing social compact between those individuals providing health care and those consuming those services. At its very core, the changing relationship between clinicians and the patients and families they serve has produced significant "dis-ease" in both groups, with growing concerns about whether the American health-care system will continue to support several popular features of the ACA, such as guaranteed issue whereby preexisting conditions do not prevent participation in health insurance plans, and how to provide dependent coverage for children on their parents' policies until age twenty-six. More specifically, the debate centering on repealing and replacing the Affordable Care Act involves a core question of whether health-care coverage is a "right" for all Americans or whether it should it remain a "privilege" for protected groups receiving financial support to offset the personal monetary impact on those fortunate enough to have medical insurance. Caught squarely in the cross hairs of this debate is the dyad of those who provide and those who consume health-care services, leading to erosion of trust between these two highly invested parties; greater degrees of job dissatisfaction and burnout among highly dedicated physicians, nurses, pharmacists, therapists, and other front-line practitioners; and dramatic confusion about how health-care consumers should access and benefit from a health system of growing complexity.

Since health-care experiences are some of the most personal of all encounters, it is of utmost importance to understand the human impact resulting from the myriad changes to the delivery landscape directly created by modifications to care practices that have arisen from legislative policy, business practices, and legal interventions. In subsequent chapters, this book will review the changes to this country's health-care system that have arisen during the past thirty years, and it will also focus on the social compact created when the health delivery system has been put under great strain from these structural changes created by health-care policies and a changing social hierarchy. As the United States moves forward with its next health-care delivery system reinvention, the changes that care providers and consumers will experience need to be well understood to avoid the unanticipated consequences that will negatively impact the lives of millions of Americans.

As a people, Americans are largely independent, autonomous, proud, and individualistic, sharing a common belief that each person should be responsible for decisions that drive the health status of an individual and the selection of health-care services being sought. The choice of one's habits, geographic location, food and drink selection, exercise, and many additional social determinants are all generally free from administrative restrictions. The sum of these individual decisions regarding health and disease then influences the political landscape directly, driving policy recommendations that are based on the effectiveness of health-care services and the cost of those services. Compared to other industrialized nations where a more egalitarian view of a "shared health-care destiny" drives population-focused policy decisions that define the ways in which payment is provided for services provided, this country's populace is far more insulated from the true costs of health care given the nature of the insurance system that has evolved. The financial impact that each American citizen makes by consuming more health services per capita than his or her Canadian and European counterparts translates into the much higher aggregated health-care costs seen in this country. In response, the United States health-care budget is growing at an alarming rate without commensurate improvement in the quality of life realized by many Americans. Any effort to provide health-care services for everyone in the nation is offset by the financial realities of how such spending growth will compromise the federal budget and its ability to sustain other public goods and services, such as the military, national infrastructure improvements, and education.

Dating from the 1940s proposals of President Harry S. Truman to the 1990s proposals of President William Jefferson Clinton and Hillary Clinton, federal policies that emphasize provision of health care as part of America's moral commitment to its citizens have all collapsed when faced with the financial pressures in play at the time. Many special-interest groups directly benefit from the health-care financing system currently in place, including physicians, hospitals, pharmaceutical companies, suppliers of durable medical equipment, and the insurers themselves. In addition, those who receive coverage as part of a protected class in society, such as Medicare and Medicaid recipients, those with employer-sponsored health plans, and those with exceptional wealth who self-fund their private insurance premiums, benefit from the coverage they receive and from political structures that reward the tax treatment of the premiums being paid by employers on their behalf. Expansion of insurance coverage to address the health-care needs of those who earn too much to qualify for Medicaid and too little to purchase insurance out-of-pocket presents financial challenges for a federal budget that is already straining from its current debt, politicized by a general disdain for implementing austerity measures or rationing care.

While many Americans routinely experience the "best" of the US health-care system, sometimes with miraculous outcomes, some segments of American society access fewer health-care services, resulting in lower degrees of overall health, produced by faulty care processes and access deficiencies that remain largely underfunded. In the end, the uneven nature of health outcomes resulting from disproportionate access and treatment inequality leaves a growing minority of Americans in a position of declining health and shorter life-span, with resultant complex social issues that magnify their underlying health concerns.[1] This struggle to "win as individuals" at the expense of a growing population of underserved differentiates the nature of the American health-care system from delivery systems found in other industrialized countries. The American health-care financing system has been perfectly designed to deliver health outcomes that are irregular and inferior when compared to other nations who "win as a group" because of more comprehensive public-payer systems that address the integrated solutions needed to favorably impact medical and social health conditions of an entire population.

Further complicating this country's issues of uneven access to care services for underinsured people is the issue of unbridled overutilization for those who are well insured. The pressure of rising costs of medications, devices, and services then puts further pressure on the practices of those involved in providing care. As part of a professional team, clinicians are charged with the burden

---

1 *World Health Statistics 2016: Monitoring Health for the SDGs Annex B: Tables of Health Statistics by Country, WHO Region and Globally,* World Health Organization, accessed May 2, 2017, http://www.who.int/gho/publications/world_health_statistics/2016/Annex_B/en/.

of acting on behalf of those whom they serve.[2] This fiduciary role is the cornerstone of professionalism where providers are expected to act first and foremost on what is best for an individual patient. But clinicians are frequently being asked to choose between exposing an already overburdened health-care financing system and the improved health outcomes that can be gained when providing additional services for an individual.

There also exists growing tension between provider groups attempting to create the greatest degree of health per dollar spent and the consumers they serve who are attempting to reduce the impact of health-care costs on their personal budgets. This schism has fundamentally changed the social compact between those providing care and those receiving care, resulting in a system of care delivery that is less fulfilling to all parties involved. Health-care professionalism has historically been able to meet the strategic goals defined by those providing financing, but the obligations of a treating practitioner are now being strained significantly by external parties such as federal policy makers and insurers who autonomously define health benefit structures and pricing. This new role for health-care professionals has produced significant emotional stress on the very people charged with designing strategies that promote better health for both individuals and entire populations needing care.

A recent report from the *Journal of the American Medical Association* (*JAMA*) cited that roughly $3.2 trillion is being spent annually on health-care services in the United States, making the American health-care system the fifth-largest economy in the world.[3] Placed in context, the most recent budget for our country's Department of Defense was just under $600 billion. Another report from *JAMA* that tracked the spending on personal health care and public health services for more than fifteen years demonstrated the significant personal pressure felt by clinicians as they struggle to provide services of high quality and safety for a population of people with increasing demands for medical services.[4] For

---

2 D. Sokol, *A Guide to the Hippocratic Oath*, BBC News, October 26, 2008, accessed May 17, 2017, http://news.bbc.co.uk/2/hi/7654432.stm.

3 E. J. Emanuel, "How Can the United States Spend Its Health Care Dollars Better?," *Journal of the American Medical Association* 316, no. 24 (2016): 2604–2606.

4 J. L. Dieleman et al., "US Spending on Personal Health Care and Public Health, 1996–2013," *Journal of the American Medical Association* 316, no. 24 (2016): 2627–2646.

the year 2013 alone, the United States spent approximately $2.4 trillion on health-care services, translating to $9,086 per person per year and accounting for 17 percent of the total US economy.[5] As a percentage of the gross domestic product (GDP), the United States spent approximately 50 percent more than any other industrialized nation but suffered from significant quality defects with outcomes for treating chronic conditions, childhood obesity, and infant mortality, which were all worse than those of other countries. Federal health programs dealing with public health issues (funded through the United States Health and Human Services [HHS], the Centers for Disease Control [CDC], Substance Abuse and Mental Health Services Administration [SAMSA], and the Food and Drug Administration [FDA]) consumed only a small fraction of the health-care dollars spent, while treatment of disease, much of which was preventable, consumed the lion's share on acute medical and surgical services. Personal health spending increased for 143 of the 155 diseases studied during the period 1996–2013, with the top three conditions being medical diseases with a clinical course that could largely have been favorably modified by more timely interventions. Diabetes mellitus, ischemic heart disease, and low back and neck pain accounted for nearly $300 billion in expenditures, with diabetes and back pain being among the five diseases with fastest-accelerating rates of health-care spending.

Before the Affordable Care Act, many Americans were excluded from health insurance coverage due to the presence of preexisting conditions, and the overall cost of care for these conditions escalated as individuals postponed care and then sought care at high-cost locations such as emergency departments and urgent-care centers. With this shift in primary-care service delivery sites, consumer value also dropped as efficiency in services delivered suffered in care-delivery sites that were not designed to care for chronic conditions. Although global spending for office-based services has now eclipsed inpatient-care spending because of efforts to reduce uncompensated care delivered in the highest-overhead sites, the fastest rates of growth in health-care spending

---

5 D. Morgan, "US Health-Care Spending Is High. Results Are…Not So Good," *CNBC Health Care*, October 8, 2015, accessed May 15, 2017, http://www.cnbc.com/2015/10/08/us-health-care-spending-is-high-results-arenot-so-good.html.

remain in emergency-department settings, where chronic-disease care planning is virtually nonexistent. These observations have led many to promote solutions that either markedly restrict access to care or reduce the per-unit reimbursement for services rendered at these high-cost sites of service. The net result of these changes has been a deepening chasm between health-care provider teams and health-care consumers.

With such a strain experienced from the proposed health-care financing solutions, one needs first to explore what separates the goals of the American health-care financing system from the systems that support the rest of the industrialized western world. In part, the "rugged individualism" created by the very birth of the United States has contributed to a market-driven system that rewards survival of the fittest. This is in significant contrast to other countries where societal norms reflect policy decisions that reinforce the "good of the whole and of the many."

One example that highlights the policy-promoted utilization differences between the US health-care delivery system and that of other industrialized states is the approach to the diagnosis and treatment of simple headache. While significant clinical evidence has been offered to American health professionals to help in their efforts to diagnose the cause of headache and provide effective and efficient treatment planning, the diagnostic approach to this clinical condition remains highly variable. Several health-care guidelines have been developed to assist in the longitudinal approach to testing, but if a patient in a resource-rich location in the United States presents with a headache, he or she will likely access many of health care's finest and most expensive technologies. These services will likely include a referral to an urgent-care center or an emergency room for initial evaluation, followed by completion of a diverse panel of blood and urine tests, a CAT scan of the brain to rule out anatomic causes of pain such as a brain tumor, and then a clinic referral to a neurologist. These services, delivered over the span of a few short hours, result in a health-care invoice that runs into the tens of thousands of dollars. This exact care plan will be repeated as often as necessary by teams of urgent-care and emergency-care providers needing to make certain that nothing has been missed previously or has developed suddenly in the interim, even if the time between headaches is only a few days and there has been no trauma or other medical condition present.

The same scenario plays out quite differently in other nations where a patient with a headache is seen by a primary care practitioner in an office setting where a careful history and physical exam are performed and where the clinician is familiar with the patient from previous visits. A simple set of tests may follow, or the provider may render a "most probable diagnosis" with appropriate therapeutic options offered and follow-up instructions given and executed by the affected individual. Should the headache not respond to initial therapy, the person is more thoroughly evaluated using a stepwise approach, with fully appropriate recommendations as outlined in evidence-based literature. The latter approach has the benefit of consuming health-care services in a more strategic fashion and generates a treatment plan that is rated as successful by both the provider and consumer of services, even as both parties acknowledge that a degree of uncertainty is inherent in this approach.

No single successful model for health-care financing has been yet devised, although the past thirty years has revealed the best of American ingenuity in trying to solve this thorny issue. Perhaps no other industry touches so many people in such a personal way as health care, and each decision made regarding the mechanism by which health care is reimbursed brings with it a visceral array of positive and negative responses. As we move toward a solution to equitably address the health-care needs of an entire population, it becomes important first to understand the solutions that have already been offered, so that we can learn from these efforts and design a delivery system that is sustainable and affordable.

George Santayana said that those who cannot remember the past are destined to repeat it,[6] so it becomes essential to understand the successes and failures of those well-intentioned individuals who came before us. The goal remains to promote policies that support a fair and reasonable reimbursement system to pay for needed health-care services for as many Americans as

---

6 George Santayana, *The Life of Reason: The Phases of Human Progress, Vol. 1, Reason in Common Sense* (Project Gutenberg, 1905).

possible and at a reasonable price that drives high-value health-care decisions. As health-care spending continues to skyrocket, one cannot underestimate the importance of establishing a payment mechanism that will maintain the best parts of the existing health-care system without bankrupting the nation. Before examining specific historical proposals, it is first important to establish the answer to a question that has plagued this country for years: is health care a right, or is it a privilege?

Three

Is Health Care a Right or a Privilege?

With every health-care reform proposal comes the question of whether health care for Americans should be viewed as a "right" for all people or a "privilege" for those who can afford it. In a recent debate, the idea that basic health-care services should be viewed as an essential right for all Americans was contrasted against a view that these services should not be forced on any of this country's citizens.[7] The argument against health care as a right centers on a conservative principle that while the framers of the Constitution focused on life, liberty, and justice, they did not mandate access to health-care services as a right for all Americans. From a viewpoint that individual liberties trump all, operating in a free-market system that encourages personal responsibility and limited government, some advocate that comprehensive health-care coverage is not guaranteed simply by citizenship. The federal government has already defined certain entitlement programs that provide for basic needs such as food and housing for most Americans. The federal budget currently provides some funding for health-care services for the elderly, poor, and disabled, but expanding health-care coverage for all Americans would create a significant

---

7 M. Gallagher and S. Hanoura, "Is Healthcare a Right?," *PBS Newshour Extra*, accessed May 18, 2017, http://www.pbs.org/newshour/extra/student_voices/debating-health-care-right-america/.

negative impact on this country's economy. In short, the "good of the many" would need to be balanced against "the benefit to the few."

The counterpoint to this argument is related to the beneficence of the American social structure, where deference is given to the needs of all Americans as part of our jointly held cultural bonds. Condoning a system of health-care financing that condemns a group of citizens to a lower quality of life, leading some Americans to suffer premature death as a result of limited access to a set of standard health-care services, is not generally accepted as a core American principle. Those who believe that access to basic health-care services is a right typically view these services as inherent to membership in a society that embraces social justice for all, and that committing a person to a life with unchecked illness based solely on that person's ability to pay runs contrary to the ideal that life is precious to all humans.

As previously discussed, the foundational principle of rugged American individualism expressed by this country's citizens has traditionally led to a view of "winning as individuals," doing so at the expense of a growing population of less fortunate. This approach also differentiates the nature of payment for health-care services found in the American health-care system from other industrialized nations who "win as a group" when they provide health-care coverage for everyone through taxation. Citizens from these nations benefit from comprehensive public payment systems that cover the integrated medical and social health-care needs of an entire population.

Complicating the issue of providing health care for all Americans is the impact already being seen from a system that provides uneven access to care services. This "underutilization of health services" contrasts with a second issue of health-care services misuse called "overutilization of health services," where financial rewards are paid to health-care providers who excessively prescribe health-care services that are of marginal value to a health-care consumer. This uneven prescribing of scarce health-care services creates pressure on those involved with providing care to dole out services with an eye on how their pattern of ordering services may be contributing to a runaway federal health-care budget. As part of a health-care delivery team, all clinicians are charged with the burden of acting on the best benefit of those they serve. This fiduciary role is the cornerstone of professionalism in which providers are expected to act first and foremost on the best behalf of a patient.[8] When viewed through the lens of the crisis seen in this county for financing health care, clinicians are frequently being asked to choose between compounding the problems of an already overburdened health-care financing system and losing the benefit gained by providing additional services for an individual. The conflict between acting on the best behalf of those they serve versus the implied role of regulating health-care spending has begun to strain the intimate relationship between doctors and patients.

Before drawing the conclusion that access to good health care is a right or a privilege for everyone in this country, one needs first to explore the many inputs into a health-care delivery system that come from the growing number of participants in the American health-care experience. How does this country's consumption of health-care dollars per capita compare to the rest of the industrialized Western world, and how does the value obtained from these investments compare to countries that have adopted schemes to finance alternative approaches? Are the investments being made to deliver the high-cost health services in the United States translating into an improved health status that justifies how those dollars are being appropriated? Is the concept of value, equating the degree to which the health status of a population improves from incremental spending, playing a significant role in the proposed policies that produce the profound economic impact felt by all Americans? To answer these questions, some understanding of the care delivery system in which this spending exists needs to be understood, along with the trade-offs that will arise from any change to that system. Kotter's change model helps us better understand the many and varied attempts to change such a large-scale system of health-care delivery, focusing on the inherent resistance to change in a complex system that produces significant sociocultural and financial impacts on a daily basis.[9]

---

8 Medical definition of Hippocratic Oath, MedicineNet.com, accessed May 17, 2017, http://www.medicinenet.com/script/main/art.asp?articlekey=20909.

9 "Kotter's 8-Step Change Model: Implementing Change Powerfully and Successfully," *MindTools*, accessed May 22, 2017, https://www.mindtools.com/pages/article/newPPM_82.htm.

Whenever one considers a stable system that is resistant to change, one needs to consider the answer to the question "What's in it for me?" for each subpopulation engaged in using that system. The system is seen at times as "too big to fail" due to its significant impact not only on the federal budget but also from the notion that every dollar spent on health care is also a dollar that contributes to the nation's gross domestic product. The thorny and interwoven nature of production and consumption creates intermediate and incomplete outcomes that are often quite opaque and difficult to interpret. Health-care service providers have grown to understand the implications of current systems of payment for service delivery, since delivery of those services is directly tied to personal revenue enhancement. Providers have developed expertise in generating a handsome living from controlling the delivery of health-care services, since they directly influence the means of production of those services. The imperfect market is created when health-care providers have access to information on effectiveness and efficiency of services that is not readily available to those consuming care, coupled with a provider's ability to order tests and perform procedures with relatively little direct oversight.

Complicating this imperfect market further is the uncertainty that comes when providers deal with the human substrate that is their patient population, and when health-care decisions are made with little individual precision and ineffective customization. Frequently driven by a narrow viewpoint of only the provider's previous experience with similar situations, decisions are imperfect from the outset. It is an oversimplification to simply blame health-care providers for health-care spending excesses given many other confounders arising from the myriad groups who benefit directly from the production of health services. Hospitals, medical insurers, suppliers, new retail entrants into the health-care delivery system, and even those who occupy positions of leadership to support these systems have become direct beneficiaries of a delivery system that brings rewards to those who are only peripherally involved. Since total health-care spending is a product of two key variables that include the cost of each unit of service delivered multiplied by the number of units of service provided, the issue of utilization of services lies prominently on those ordering those services. Whenever the unit cost of services is decreased, such as when the government or private insurers modify a fee schedule, the provider's overall economic advantage can be maintained simply by generating more services.

For supporting industries such as health insurance companies, any increase in global spending arising from a group of people insured is passed on as an increase in health insurance premiums the following year. By passing on the costs of the medical losses experienced, insurers can maintain necessary financial reserves for future payments while also covering the cost of the administrative load (overhead) of running the insurance business. Included in the administrative load of insurers are executive salaries and benefits, a key financial issue of concern for many Americans attempting to secure a better status of health while also managing the spiraling costs of expensive health insurance. For every dollar given to health insurance executives that comes from health insurance premiums, a dollar is unavailable for health-care services. Many health-care consumers who have experienced significant increases in their health insurance premiums have equated exorbitant compensation of insurance executives with trends of lower levels of health-care benefits being made available to them at even higher prices. From a recent report, the top thirty-three executives of Blue Cross and Blue Shield Plans received $102 million in total compensation to help administer those plans, and compensation formulas are now being monitored by the Securities and Exchange Commission as of 2017.[10]

In 1996, as I was completing a master's degree in administrative medicine, I accepted a position at a provider-owned health plan in northern Indiana as the chief medical officer to help administer medical benefits found in the plan's Certificate of Coverage and to create a quality improvement program. Having previously helped start such a plan in Iowa, I was intrigued with the possibility of helping coordinate benefits for thousands of people who chose to access health insurance coverage directly through a health plan operating at a very thin margin. With direct access to provider-owners of the plan and with

---

10 "The AIS Report on Blue Cross and Blue Shield Plans," *AIS Health* 14, no. 10 (October 2015), accessed May 22, 2017, https://aishealth.com/archive/nblu1015-01.

greater amounts of the premium dollar being spent directly on patient care, this great experiment in insurance was earning rave reviews from consumers, providers, and businesses.

Moving from my clinical practice of nephrology and transplant medicine in Iowa, I found the leaders of the Indiana health plan to be committed not only to the sound business principles required to run a finely tuned business, but also to patient-centered principles guiding innovative products and services that were being offered to patients. Constant communication with patients, doctors, and hospitals gave me the comfort of knowing that the medical needs of beneficiaries were being met, and there was little of the premium dollar left unaccounted for in what was labeled the "medical loss ratio," reflecting the percentage of premium being spent on health-care services. The plan had grown significantly, providing insurance coverage for over 175,000 people, with careful attention to the quality of claims payment, interpretation of benefits, and network relations with doctors and hospitals that created a very successful business model for insurance. As a provider-owned plan with rules promulgated by the Indiana Department of Insurance, the health plan continued to meet its reserve requirements, largely due to the sweat equity invested by the provider-owners of the plan and through careful care coordination efforts perfected by the plan's medical management strategies.

In 1981, the Indiana General Assembly created a not-for-profit association to provide a safety net for citizens unable to secure insurance coverage in the private insurance marketplace, serving as an alternative to MediGap coverage for those under age sixty-five.[11] The program, called the Indiana Comprehensive Health Insurance Association (ICHIA), was funded in part by high-risk individuals seeking coverage, with the remaining 50 percent of the costs paid by the State of Indiana, shared with all health insurers operating in the state. Remaining solvent for nearly twenty years, the state-administered program plan began to develop significant financial pressures as more people

---

11 "Final Program Budget Submission," Indiana Comprehensive Health Insurance Association, December 12, 2013, accessed April 2, 2017, https://secure.in.gov/sba/files/BC_Hearing_2012_ICHIA_Program_Overview.pdf.

required coverage through the ICHIA program, and those who were seeking coverage had significant medical complexity with high care costs. Recognizing that the program funding had to be enhanced, the insurance commissioner proposed a special ICHIA tax to be paid by all health maintenance organizations (HMOs) in Indiana, placing greater hardship on plans that were operating at very thin financial margins.

Over the course of two years after the implementation of the new ICHIA tax, the provider-owned health plan that had been so well accepted by patients and providers alike began to suffer financial hardships, while other higher-margin health insurance plans such as Blue Cross Blue Shield had reserves deep enough to weather the financial storm of such a tax. A capital call was made to the owners of the provider-based plan, and a decision was made to strategically exit from the insurance marketplace given what appeared to be even larger financial commitments needed in the future. Individuals and employer-based plan beneficiaries had fewer choices when the provider-based plan closed for business, and health insurance premiums in the marketplace increased significantly, allowing larger health plans to profit from their high-margin model.

For suppliers, great economic benefit is realized whenever new indications for a drug or device are promoted or whenever a less costly medication or device is replaced by another that is deemed to be superior because of advances in health-care technology. One example of the impact from drug replacement is in the treatment of immunologically active diseases such as psoriasis, for which an inexpensive topical medication that has been used successfully for years has been replaced by very expensive injectable immunotherapy. Highly touted in direct-to-consumer television advertisements as being markedly superior to previous therapies, immunotherapy regimens can result in thousands of dollars of additional spending on medications each year. Although some insurance plans restrict access to these advanced treatments in first-line strategies, suppliers continue to extend patents on other expensive medications by slightly modifying how those drugs are administered. Alternative indications for medications can also help big pharmaceutical companies preserve patent protections and company profits while defraying the sunk research and development costs.

Those who consume health-care services also play a direct role in the rapid rise in health-care costs, as individuals who are significantly insulated from the costs of care through health insurance continue to demand tests and treatments of marginal utility. These "covered lives" follow traditional economic incentives to consume health-care services that have been promoted in the marketplace, since they have little economic disincentive against consumption. The groups who benefit most from such arrangements are participants in employer-based health plans with significant offset to premiums paid by their employers, those who participate in veteran benefits (VA health-care services), those enrolled in Medicare (elderly and disabled) and Medicaid (below-poverty-level poor) entitlement programs, and those with no financial means to pay for health-care services, meaning that no incentive exists to them to pay for health-care services that have been delivered. These protected groups also consume health care by following traditional economic incentives, with greater numbers of health services consumed as deductibles and out-of-pocket costs are satisfied, leading to fewer expenses out of pocket toward the end of the calendar year. This consumption pattern has been demonstrated as care consumers may put off tests and treatments early in a benefit year to reduce the monetary impact of expensive services being rendered early in a calendar year. This same incentive is seen when individuals schedule tests and treatments later in the year when no additional out-of-pocket expenses will be recorded, as they have met their deductibles and copayments. This postponement of services generates some of the negative health impact that results when there are delays in treatment of chronic conditions early in a calendar year.[12] It also helps explain the increased market demand for services during November and December, when surgical volumes for elective procedures, such as tonsillectomy and placement of drainage tubes in the ears of pediatric patients, are highly disproportionate compared to earlier months of the year.

With a US health-care system that has been perfectly constructed to benefit those producing and those consuming care, there is little impetus to change

---

12 "Dig Deep: Impacts and Implications of Rising Out-of-Pocket Health Care Costs," *Deloitte Center for Health Solutions*, accessed May 24, 2017, https://www2.deloitte.com/content/dam/Deloitte/us/Documents/life-sciences-health-care/us-lchs-dig-deep-hidden-costs-112414.pdf.

the rules of engagement in how services are designed, deployed, and paid for. The impact of this "perfectly designed system," however, is felt most by those who do not fall into one of the protected groups mentioned previously. The losers in this economic quagmire are those individuals who are nonqualifiers for supported services, such as those who earn too much to qualify for Medicaid services but earn too little to purchase their own health insurance. The rapid rise in numbers of nonqualifiers has been complicated by less adequate employer-based insurance coverage with the rise of defined contribution and high-deductible health plans. These insurance structures allow individuals to purchase insurance protection against the risk of catastrophic events but may delay or defer services for other chronic but not life-threatening conditions. This group of uninsured and underinsured has been growing steadily so that by 2009, nearly 17 percent of Americans had no form of private or government insurance program coverage, and the Congressional Budget Office found that nearly half of all Americans were without some form of coverage for at least a portion of a year.[13]

Not only do individuals from this underinsured group have significant financial obstacles looming just around the corner should a medical catastrophe strike, they are also placed at risk by the absence of a personal savings account following the economic downturn of 2008. The final nail in the coffin for this group is the lack of political representation that could assist them by providing a voice for protection of funding for health-care services they need to retain personal economic solvency. The nature of politics centers on protecting those with the loudest voices, and at the heart of this moral dilemma is that those most in need of medical services have the least political clout. With little hope of overcoming their position of disenfranchisement, they rely on hard work and good fortunes to prevent financial disaster. It is estimated that three in five bankruptcies are due to an inability to pay medical bills, and 20 percent of American adults struggle to pay for needed

---

13 Congressional Budget Office, *Methods for Analyzing Health Insurance Coverage*, accessed May 24, 2017, https://www.cbo.gov/topics/health-care/methods-analyzing-health-insurance-coverage.

medical services.[14] In the same article, Christina LaMontagne, vice president of *NerdWallet*, provider of financial advice and user-friendly decision support tools to consumers, states that twenty-five million people hesitate to take their medications as a personal financial strategy aimed at controlling their medical costs. The burden of rapidly rising health-care costs far outweighs the impact seen from proposed faulty financial management by poor people, since many examples also exist of middle-class Americans being financially overwhelmed when a catastrophic illness or injury arises.

Shifting to the macroeconomic impact on the US economy, health-care costs continue to place significant strain on a federal budget that is already stretched from commitments to improve and enhance infrastructure, provide military funding, and meet the national security concerns of a tense and complex world. As both the utilization and cost of medical services continue to rise at a breakneck rate, the federal budgetary impact realized from health-care spending grows even more worrisome in America when compared to the cost impact felt by other industrialized nations. In 1970, the United States, Canada, Sweden, and Denmark spent roughly the same percentage of their federal budget on health care, approximately 7 percent of the gross domestic product.[15] In response to a free-market solution for health-care funding in the United States, this country has seen annual growth rates in spending over the past thirty years that have drastically exceeded the next most costly industrialized nation.

In addition to excess service consumption seen in the United States, the 50 percent higher spending is magnified by the impact from covering social-services issues currently being paid through medical insurance. While many other industrialized nations split social-services costs from true medical-care spending, the United States addresses many social issues using health-care dollars. An example of how medical-service dollars are used for social-services

14 "Money, Cash, Throes. 643,000 Americans Go Bankrupt Each Year over Medical Bills," Snopes.com, April 22, 2016, accessed May 3, 2017, http://www.snopes.com/643000-bankruptcies-in-the-u-s-every-year-due-to-medical-bills/.

15 "A System of Health Accounts 2011, Revised Edition," *Organisation for Economic Co-Operation and Development, European Union, World Health Organization* (Paris: OECD Publishing, 2017).

needs is evident in today's opioid drug crisis. Those unfortunate individuals who are addicted to narcotics frequently visit multiple emergency departments to secure medications as part of their self-directed approach to their mental-health condition of addiction, leading to ineffective strategies for treatment and great inefficiency in care delivery. In emergency rooms across the country, stopgap measures that produce little long-term benefit are provided to individuals wrestling with a condition that would be more effectively and efficiently treated in a mental-health center. Since mental- and behavioral-health centers are often culturally and geographically separated from traditional medical sites of service, communication between medical and mental-health providers is frequently lacking, and development of a comprehensive approach to care is limited. This poorly coordinated approach leads to payment for services from health-care budgets that cover the health consequences that are direct complications arising from social-services and mental-health deficiencies.

With all the above factors in play, there is little doubt why there exists growing tension within provider groups that are attempting to create the greatest degree of health per dollar spent and those in the political and insurance sectors who are attempting to down-regulate health-care payments. This schism has also fundamentally changed the social compact between those providing care and those receiving care. Professionalism has met the strategic practicalities of health-care financing, and the fiduciary obligations of a treating practitioner are being dictated with ever-greater scrutiny by external parties such as policy makers and those in charge of determining how health benefits are structured and paid at health insurance companies. This confusing and confrontational role for health-care professionals produces a significant emotional burden on those charged with designing effective health-care strategies that promote an improved health status for individuals and populations of patients.

Even if the issues of health-care services consumption in America could be addressed by adopting a more egalitarian approach to medical decision-making, there remains the issue of growing medical complexity and consumerism in an environment where information asymmetry exists. Since health-care providers better understand the benefits and limitations of key services that are required, health-care consumers feel less empowered to participate in developing medical strategies that impact their lives. Not only has health care become more highly specialized and complex, but physical navigation through the morass of health care has become much more difficult as multiple connection points that are highly fragmented are assembled loosely as part of an "integrated" delivery network. Several new entrants into the delivery system, such as retail pharmacy and big-box medical clinics, are not directly integrated with health systems, delivering piecemeal services that may be more easily accessed at a lower cost but suffer from a lack of a comprehensive approach to testing and treatment. A common example is when a person seeks an influenza vaccination, and delivery of that service at a retail pharmacy may cost less than services found at a physician office. While less expensive, these services are not integrated with a patient's longitudinal medical record, creating an environment where the health-care consumer is the responsible agent for coordination of services. Consumers must then inform their treatment team when any adjustment is made to medications or diet, or when tests have been performed.

The health-care delivery structures of today are "systems without systemness," which should not be surprising when one considers the many inputs that have been created to address a consumer's desire to seek high-value health care. This approach also places increased personal responsibility for care coordination on the consumer, requiring individuals to serve as their own care navigator across multiple disparate sites of service. The question of whether the next step in the evolution of health-care delivery systems will yield better outcomes when compared to historic care delivery experiences is currently unknown, but complex changes seen in today's systems have certainly strained the relationship between those delivering care and those receiving care. Whether health care is actually a right for all Americans or simply a privilege to be experienced by a few protected classes is important in the context of federal and state health-care policies, but as these new policies have stimulated experiments in health-care service delivery and funding, there is a recognition that the bond between clinicians and their communities has been weakened. As this relationship continues to dissolve and health care is viewed as "just another business," providers and consumers are beginning to realize the negative unintended consequences found in a health-care team that has not lost the passion to care for and about patients. This personal passion for care delivery is limited to care that can be delivered at well-defined sites of service and provided by health-care workers who are limited by the number of shifts they are scheduled.

What the ultimate result will be from this new delivery system and its new incentives is unknown, but it is most likely that Americans will experience a health-care delivery system where coordination of services is lacking, and trust will be diminished. The next few years, filled with innovative approaches, will define the health-care services that can be afforded and the groups that can receive them, diminishing the importance of an argument about whether health care is a right or a privilege. As this distinction falls in prominence for most everyone except policy makers, payment practices will drive the answer to this question, leaving the American health-care landscape permanently changed, impacting the number of individuals fortunate enough to secure health insurance coverage for essential services. Not only will policy and payment models drive access to key services, they will also help redefine the relationship between those providing care and those receiving care.

Key Points to Master From Chapter 3

- Debate on whether access to health care is a "right" or a "privilege" has been at the root of sixty years of health care policy funding considerations.
- Many factors determine the "value" of health care in an imperfect marketplace, with health care providers, consumers, payers, and suppliers all playing key roles.
- Kotter's model for understanding how change occurs in complex adaptive systems helps us appreciate the many agendas that need to be addressed before longer term and meaningful improvements in health care financing can be implemented.
- Three of five bankruptcies in the United States result from unpaid medical bills, and 20% of Americans struggle to pay for medical services. A lack of health insurance, loss of savings, underemployment, and an escalating cost of health care all contribute to significant financial stress experienced by nearly half of all Americans.
- Health care policies will define the mechanisms of payment for health care services and the groups of people who can access those services; those same policies will dramatically affect the strength of the compact between providers and consumers.

Section 2
The New Order

INTRODUCTION TO SECTION 2

The slightly tilted black fedora and narrow gray lines superimposed on the dark-blue suit made the short and bespectacled Dr. Abraham Tobas easily recognized as he meandered down the hospital's hallways, popping in and out of patient rooms. One of the first learned scholars I met in medical school, Dr. Tobas was a fixture at Iowa Lutheran Hospital in Des Moines, having been a diabetes specialist on staff for nearly fifty years. Following his training at the Joslin Clinic in Boston, Tobas had built one of the earliest endocrinology practices in the Midwest, hiring his wife as his only office employee. Having been trained in the meticulous care of diabetics by precisely measuring each of his patient's food items to the exact ounce, Dr. Tobas could be seen in the hospital kitchen peering over the top of his gold wire-rimmed glasses measuring his patient's food portions on a small scale and recording these weights into a small black notebook he carried with him at all times. Sending the food trays on their way to his patients, he would then quickly disappear to meet his patients and supervise their regular insulin administration at least four times each day.

I first met the diabetes specialist when he strolled into the emergency room late one evening to chat with his longtime friend and colleague, Dr. Donald Nord. The funny and cantankerous Nord, a primary-care physician himself, often chided Tobas about who possessed the greater knowledge regarding the latest discoveries in diabetes care. In return, Dr. Tobas frequently kidded Nord about his Norwegian heritage, and the two men could be seen sharing a hearty laugh well into the night in the emergency department. As part of my education, the elder diabetologist took me under his wing to make certain that I gained an appreciation for the great men and women of medicine who had come before me. Weaving in the stories of sacrifice and devotion to patients that had become the trademark of the physicians of his era, he also gave me bits of medical history that provided context to my chosen profession.

One such story related to the invention of the stethoscope, which had been initially developed to ease the anxiety and tension that filled the room when a male physician placed his ear directly on a female patient's chest to hear heart sounds. After a French physician, Dr. Rene Laennec, became uncomfortable at the prospect of directly listening to the heart of a young woman, he rolled up a magazine and placed it between his ear and the woman's chest. Hearing heart sounds even better using this primitive device, he proclaimed that he had developed the first instrument to better auscultate the heart. He called this new contraption a "stethoscope"; it resembled the ear trumpets prevalent in France at the time, which provided amplification of ambient sounds such as voice and music, thereby promoting better hearing. Over the next fifty years, many iterations of the listening device were used, and in the mid-1850s, Dr. George Philip Cammann perfected the first design to be made commercially available.

As Dr. Tobas told the story, he reflected on his own interest in innovation of medical devices, and he confided that he had constructed his own stethoscope based on the original design of Cammann. Piecing together the precise length of rubber tubing as described by early researchers, Tobas glued a chrome-plated spring-loaded binaural chest piece to the rubber tubes and then used specially constructed soft earpieces that were sealed to the chest piece binaural using violin bowstring wax. The entire device was then connected to a stethoscope listening head composed of both a diaphragm that transmitted high-frequency noises and a conical tube that was used to detect rumbling murmurs and other lower-frequency sounds. The stethoscope listening device had been perfected by Sir William Osler, one of the founders of Johns Hopkins Hospital, and Dr. Tobas had designed his customized listening device based on specifications that were meticulously researched and unparalleled in their simplicity. As a "grand old gentleman of medicine," his journey to perpetually improve the practice of health care was obvious, and I felt privileged to personally witness it during our encounters. One of the greatest gifts I received when I completed medical school was a personally constructed stethoscope made by Dr. Tobas that I carried every day until I retired from clinical practice.

Sitting with a very elderly Abraham Tobas at his bedside as he was dying, I was astounded that he continued to educate me about the signs and symptoms of his clinical condition to help imprint them into my diagnostic repertoire, while also reminding me about the grace and courage that patients possess as human beings as they approach the end of their lives. Lessons such as these, taught by the great men and women of medicine, were transferred as part of a "rite of passage" that helped the youngest physicians in training better understand the tremendous responsibility that was being given to them, and helped clarify the unique privilege granted me to interact compassionately with people when they are most vulnerable at the end of their lives.

Today's health-care system is much more complex than when Dr. Tobas was helping create a learning environment for young minds. With daily stresses related to the time pressures of keeping to a schedule in the office or clinic, reimbursement stresses defining the solvency of medical practices, new administrative burdens created by health insurance companies, the frustration of dealing with federal and state government regulations, the new requirements of public reporting of quality and safety outcomes, and greater demands being placed on health-care providers by care consumers, it is no wonder that some of the joy has been lost from the practice of providing health care while attempting to retain the best of a caring environment. Even the perspective of providing care to vulnerable people as a privilege has begun to erode, as health-care providers are beginning to see themselves more as "shift workers" than health-care professionals who are committed to providing an irreplaceable service for their community. With more entrants into the care-delivery space arriving every year, including retail pharmacy, big-box stores, and freestanding clinics delivering alternative and complementary services, these interruptions have strained the once-strong bond that has previously unified practitioner and patient.

It is important to gain a better understanding of the roles of the new participants in today's health-care experience to see how they may all best interface with one another. We are currently at the beginning of a grand experiment to reimagine a new world of health-care delivery in which multiple voices and viewpoints need to be balanced on behalf of those being served. If we can better understand how the participants might integrate with one another, we may be able to begin a dialogue about the best way to provide access to care for all people while reducing the significant financial burden being placed on health insurers and on federal and state budgets. At the heart of this understanding is a desire to maintain one of the most important aspects of the care experience, that of the provider-patient relationship, which is essential to maximize the effectiveness of care and to promote satisfaction with the care process itself. As a long-standing participant and advocate of such a relationship, I am continuously driven to reintroduce joy into the health-care delivery experience and to strengthen the bond that has begun to erode between those providing care and those receiving it. Remembering an adage given to me by Dr. Tobas when he challenged me to always remember that "there is no care without caring," I refuse to give up on the significant benefits and beauty that can arise when people delivering care and people receiving care are unified in purpose, respectful of each other's role, and focused on the end product of restoring health and well-being.

Four

The New Health-Care Delivery Team

The new health delivery system paradigm calls for provision of medical services that are of highest quality and safety at a lower cost (producing high value) by aligning and integrating treatment teams and continuum partners (network development) and leveraging these capabilities to drive differentiation and viability in the changing health-care environment (enhanced financial outcomes). Current health-care systems are viewed as "focused factories" that concentrate on narrow interventions, focusing on shorter-term progress using a disease-based approach, and they have component provider elements that are not strategically well aligned with either their peers or the specific goals expressed by the people they serve. What all participating parties are looking for is an integrated and interdependent set of practice units that are accountable for the total care of a person, focusing on the longer-term well-being of health-care consumers with progress and success defined by the outcomes that arise from an entire episode of care or a lifetime of wellness. The simplicity of a single physician providing care for all members of his or her community has been replaced by a highly complex constellation of care providers who appear to be unaffiliated and incompletely aware of what each is doing on behalf of a person struggling to attain a greater health status.

A former colleague once told me that the needs of people interacting with the health-care industrial complex are quite simple:[16]

- If a person is healthy, he or she just wants to remain healthy.
- If a person in ill or injured, he or she just wants to get better.
- If a person needs admission to a hospital, he or she just wants to feel safe and return home in as close to his or her original health status as possible or improved from baseline.
- When a person interacts with a health-care provider, he or she wants to be treated kindly and with respect.

Complexity of health-care experiences has exploded as innovative technologies challenge patients and care providers who are wrestling with advances in medical diagnostics and surgical techniques and with greater numbers of interested parties surrounding the person with illness or injury. Most of this march toward better care has been a direct benefit to the consumer of care, but it has left many patients, family members, and sometimes providers themselves in need of a course in medical literacy to determine how best to interact with such a system of care. The new medical "neighborhood" has evolved from the medical "home" of the past and now includes a host of people providing guidance and suggestions, and even a cottage industry has begun to be built around those who help coordinate care services or those who assist in "patient navigation" through the complex care experience. The set of services and care plans needing to be coordinated include those experienced in both acute and chronic care, services that promote wellness and prevention, primary and specialty care provider services, short-term and longer-term care services, and even the recently added "nontraditional" retail services being provided by large chain pharmacy and big-box retail outlets.

Assessing the success of such a system has also changed, shifting from a focus on measuring the processes of care (the set of services being provided) to a desire to concentrate on the most important person-specific outcomes that

16 Attributed to Lance Peterson, MD, clinical pathologist and infectious disease specialist at NorthShore University HealthSystem, Evanston, Illinois.

target a set of goals related to promoting, restoring, or maintaining higher degrees of health. These new goals, defined through the collaborative efforts of both the consumer and provider of care, are much more relevant, integrated, transparent, understandable, flexible, and comprehensive than previous metrics regarding the outputs of care delivery. It's no small wonder that health-care reform plans are so difficult to construct, since system goals are evolving quickly in front of the eyes of providers of care, consumers of care, payers for care, and regulators of care, with an incomplete capacity for delivering all needed services in the communities where care is experienced.

The migration from a single physician–single patient relationship has been progressive, due to the growing complexity of health-care services and the time pressures of health-care delivery. The mounting stress felt by practicing physicians has begun to take its toll not only on the historic bond between providers and consumers of care, but also on the emotional well-being of providers. A recent article outlines the many reasons for provider burnout that has resulted from mounting pressures on physicians, including narrowed insurance networks, physician employment arrangements, greater pressures to generate more "patient transactions," and reduced physician autonomy.[17] Coupling these new business practices with an ever-expanding knowledge of medicine that must be mastered, the depersonalization of the clinician-patient bond arising in part from the use of electronic health records, and public reporting of quality and safety data, providers have struggled with increasing degrees of emotional injury as their personal satisfaction with their chosen occupation dropped significantly.[18,19]

The impact from implementation of electronic health records cannot be understated given its impact on the social compact between provider and

17 T. D. Shanafelt, L. N. Dyrbye, and C. P. West, "Addressing Physician Burnout: The Way Forward," *Journal of the American Medical Association* 317, no. 9 (2017): 901–902.

18 T. D. Shanafelt, S. Boone, L. Tan, et al., "Burnout and Satisfaction with Work-Life Balance among US Physicians Relative to the General US Population," *Archives of Internal Medicine* 172, no. 18 (2012): 1377–1385.

19 T. D. Shanafelt, O. Hasan, L. N. Dyrbye, et al., "Changes in Burnout and Satisfaction with Work-Life Balance in Physicians and the General US Working Population between 2011 and 2014," *Mayo Clinic Proceedings* 90, no. 12 (2015): 1600–1613.

consumer, but also because of the personal toll it has taken in provider joy due to the time spent in maintaining the record and the new demands from after-hours asynchronous responses to patient questions that arise from the use of a patient information portal for expanded communication. One estimate of the amount of time spent in uncompensated clerical duties to support clinical encounters showed that for every hour spent in providing clinical care, nearly twice that amount of time was spent in clerical support of that care, amounting to almost half of the total workday.[20]

A recent article in the primary-care journal *Family Practice Management* explored how primary-care physicians can see greater numbers of patients in less time while providing greater care coordination if they utilize physician assistants or nurse practitioners, sometimes referred to as "extenders" of physician services.[21] This approach is largely designed to create greater system efficiency while also controlling costs, since less-trained care personnel can be used to evaluate and treat patients with relatively minor illnesses or injuries. The new care delivery team also hopes to reduce the stress that leads to burnout of primary-care physicians who have been charged with resolving a comprehensive set of cares and concerns for each patient. The emotional stresses that have emerged have left many primary-care physicians contemplating how they might retire earlier, further compromising the shrinking pool of doctors who are battling at the front lines of health care.[22,23] The call has gone out to find competent, motivated, and passionate colleagues who will step up to share the growing workload produced from greater administrative and

20 C. Sinsky, L. Colligan, L. Li, et al., "Allocation of Physician Time in Ambulatory Practice: A Time and Motion Study in 4 Specialties," *Annals of Internal Medicine* 165, no. 11 (2016): 753–760.

21 V. S. Kaprielian, J. Kase, and T. Higgins, "What Can a PA or NP Do for Your Practice?," *Family Practice Management* 24, no. 2 (2017): 19–22.

22 R. C. Rabin and Kaiser Health News, "A Growing Number of Primary-Care Doctors Are Burning Out. How Does This Affect Patients?," *The Washington Post*, March 31, 2014, accessed May 11, 2017, https://www.washingtonpost.com/national/health-science/a-growing-number-of-primary-care-doctors-are-burning-out-how-does-this-affect-patients/2014/03/31/2e8bce24-a951-11e3-b61e-8051b8b52d06_story.html?utm_term=.6fd52e6e7245.

23 F. Zenasni, E. Boujut, A. Woerner, and S. Sultan, "Burnout and Empathy in Primary Care: Three Hypotheses," *British Journal of General Practice* 62, no. 600 (2012): 346–347.

reporting burdens that have been squarely targeted to the primary-care work site.[24,25]

The evolution of the health-care treatment team of today has been created not only by the expansion of care services with additional layers of complexity but also by the ways in which that complexity has impacted the social compact for care that was in effect before the turn of the century. Despite the toll it took on personal well-being, physicians often blurred the lines between vocation and avocation as they placed themselves in a position where they created a grand bargain with their communities. In return for lifelong commitment to the community, providing access and availability twenty-four hours a day, seven days a week, and frequently fifty-two weeks each year, physicians received the trade-off of being handsomely paid and even occupying a revered place in the community's social hierarchy. Given great deference by their neighbors, physicians were trusted to provide relief to persons with illness or injury, often acting as their patients' surrogates in the decision-making practices in the era of medical paternalism, further reinforcing the dictum that a provider was placing a patients' needs above his or her own.

This organized system of care was quite understandable, and the simplicity of holding a single expert accountable for health-care decisions was appreciated by nearly every participant in the experience. Models for such trusted community patriots were everywhere, from magazine advertisements where physicians recommended specific brands of cigarettes for their patients, to medical soap operas where sage and experienced physicians provided care in their homes. Such caring environments were not dedicated specifically to an end point of curing illness, but focused more on the ways in which those providers were always present during these times of injury or illness. Approaching a model similar to clergy, the entire community benefitted from having dedicated care providers always at their disposal. Extending care practices beyond

---

24 S. Porter, "Curbing Primary Care Burnout Epidemic: Address Physician, Staff Needs First, Say Researchers," *AAFP News*, December 3, 2014, accessed May 11, 2017, http://www.aafp.org/news/practice-professional-issues/20141203annfammedburnout.html.

25 S. Okie, "Innovation in Primary Care—Staying One Step Ahead of Burnout," *New England Journal of Medicine* 359 (November 27, 2008): 2305–2309.

their small offices, these physicians were available for crises found in the hospital or a patient's home, and since these providers knew their community members well, the need for complex record keeping was minimized.

One such real-life primary-care provider was Dr. Carlton Van Natta, whose practice was viewed as a shining example of what primary care looked like in the last half of the twentieth century. Born in 1916, Dr. Van Natta frequently referred patients to me for my opinion regarding kidney disease. Whether I received a letter from him introducing a patient to me or just spoke with him in the hospital about one of his office patients, it was always obvious that he knew virtually everything about the person being sent for evaluation. He could instantly recite not only the patient's medical problem list but also the medications that he and other practitioners had prescribed, specific patient allergies, the year in which the patient met and married his or her spouse, the college destinations of the patients' children, and whether or not the person had previous scrapes with the law or marital infidelity. Van, as he was called by his colleagues, exemplified the old adage that "the best thing about a small community is that everyone knows your business, while the worst thing about a small community is that everyone knows your business." Van Natta's patients loved him, having shared their challenging medical experiences with this gentle soul whose friendly and committed nature allowed him to reach out with a gentle hand to provide comfort and support to their families. Seeing the good doctor working long hours every day, I can recall only a handful of times in my practice life that a phone call about one of his patients was ever answered by someone other than him. A slight man with thinning reddish-brown hair, Van Natta could frequently be heard whistling as he briskly walked between his car and the hospital, where he visited each of his patients every day while they were confined. Keeping up with the progress of a complicated and hospitalized patient was just one aspect of his comprehensive approach to patient care, and it was obvious that this commitment was part of his definition of how one accepted the responsibility of becoming a family physician.

Still other physicians found it necessary to take on informal assistants in their practices, particularly if the practice involved several sites of service, especially when time needed to be split between the operating room, hospital inpatient floors, and the practice office. The most clinically competent and well-liked nursing staff are frequent targets to be added to a physician practice, serving in roles that include preparing the day's clinical information such as laboratory tests or X-rays that need to be previewed, writing notes to confirm hospital documentation for reimbursement, or even answering simple questions raised by patients and their families in the physician's absence. These nurse specialists are frequently provided with on-the-job training to help round out their clinical acumen, and they help busy physicians "be in two places at one time." Quality of care is favorably influenced, since these new members of the treatment team can screen the needs of patients and discuss results of tests and treatments without the time pressures that are growing for physician providers. Reimbursement for these added services comes as part of a private employment agreement with the physician, and no additional reimbursement from private insurers or government payers is received. Some specialty nursing providers remain employed by hospitals directly to help with essential functions such as performance of preoperative history and physical examinations, to help minimize adverse safety events and to provide greater service to the physicians who schedule surgical procedures at those institutions. Still other nursing specialists serve as "navigators" to help patients and families move though the health-care experience while also coordinating the care needs of a person in the midst of a complex treatment plan being provided by multiple physicians.

In addition to the less formalized approach of clinical nurses who are hired to aid physicians, some new members of the care team are added as semiautonomous clinicians with their own professional certification. These new team members were initially labeled as "midlevel providers" or the much-maligned term "physician extenders," largely because they still required some form of physician supervision and had diminished autonomy. One type of midlevel provider, the physician assistant (PA), is nationally certified and state-licensed to perform a number of services such as conducting physical exams, ordering and interpreting tests, diagnosing illnesses, developing treatment plans, coordinating care, performing procedures, prescribing medications, engaging in clinical research, advising on preventive health care, and serving as assistants to surgeons in the operating room.[26] Typically trained for six years, these team members hold the equivalent of a master's degree, and their education mirrors what was created to provide fast-track training for physicians during World War II, when the supply of doctors was limited. The first educational program to train PAs was established in 1965, and rules to establish accreditation for primary-care physician assistants came in 1971 from the Council on Medical Education from the American Medical Association.[27] Since that time, thousands of PAs have been trained and are frequently seen by the communities they serve as the "local doctor."

Another type of midlevel provider joining the evolving health-care team, a nurse practitioner (NP), is a qualified professional who can diagnose medical problems, order treatments, perform advanced procedures, prescribe medications in some states, and make referrals for a wide range of acute and chronic medical conditions within their scope of practice.[28] In some states with a significant shortage of physicians, NPs operate without physician oversight, and many specialize to provide care for patients with a wide array of care needs such as orthopedics, surgery, oncology, pain management, dermatology, and women's health. Just as with PAs, NPs are certified nationally, and since they are licensed by states, there is some variation in the types of services they can provide, as well as the practice constraints faced by NPs who serve as independent providers of care.

The expanding set of health-care team roles has also affected physician providers, where new specialties have arisen to provide care for patients at specific sites of service. A recent Viewpoint article from the *Journal of the American Medical Association* has cited that the workforce of the future will demand clinicians who can better manage acute conditions found in the hospital setting. Treating complex medical conditions such as cancer, stroke, and

26 *Physician Associate Program: the PA Profession*, Yale School of Medicine, January 4, 2013, accessed March 14, 2017.

27 *National Commission on Certification of Physician Assistants*, accessed May 12, 2017, https://www.nccpa.net/.

28 "Definition and Characteristics of the Role," *International Council of Nurses (ICN) International Nurse Practitioner/Advanced Practice Nursing Network*, accessed March 14, 2017, http://international.aanp.org/Practice/APNRoles.

cardiac conditions have better clinical outcomes if key skills are developed and utilized by physicians whose focus is on maintaining proficiency in the use of those skills by repetitive exposure to these conditions.[29,30] Primary-care physicians have differentiated into these specialty areas as "hospitalists" (care of patients confined in acute medical-surgical areas of hospitals), "intensivists" (care provided in intensive care units), or "SNFists" (providing services in skilled nursing facilities, previously called nursing homes or long-term care facilities). Differentiation of primary-care physician roles has been cited as an improvement in the physician care model because it allows office-based clinicians to more efficiently spend time caring for outpatient conditions, reinforcing the belief that a more dedicated primary-care team can generate strategies that more completely fulfill the preventive care needs of people, resulting in greater wellness while maintaining the enhanced health status of people who are otherwise generally healthy.

Some clinicians are now being deployed within hospital sites of care in much the same way emergency medicine physicians diversified from being part-time shift workers to full-time emergency medicine specialists. Hospitalists are now in place in most hospitals, and the specialty of hospital medicine is one of the fastest-growing and most demanding of all specialties. The advantages of hospitalist care transcend the simple ability of a physician to develop comfort with an acutely ill person and to better deploy current knowledge in dealing with highly complex patients. Many hospitals also look to the hospitalist to reduce the length of hospital stays, helping create labor efficiencies that lead to better financial margins at a time when federal and private insurance has begun to reimburse on a single prospective payment rather than paying for services on a per diem (daily) basis. One additional benefit realized by hospitals employing their own physician pool is the ability to engage these well-trained physicians in focused quality and patient safety improvement projects that further enhance the clinical outcomes needed to financially profit from

29 S. H. Lipstein and A. L. Kellerman, "Workforce for 21st-Century Health and Health Care," *Journal of the American Medical Association* 316, no. 16 (2016): 1665–1666.

30 Institute of Medicine, *Regionalizing Emergency Care: Workshop Summary* (Washington, DC: National Academies Press, 2010).

new reimbursement schema that reward the "value" of services provided rather than just the number of services provided.

One active participant group that has not yet expressed full-throated enthusiasm for the new hospital-based physician practice is the patient and family dyad. When primary-care physicians, who knew a great deal about individual patients and their families, used to make hospital rounds on their own patients, an integrated and comprehensive treatment plan that fully incorporated patient preferences was relatively easy to implement. In the current model, information about patient preferences is frequently missing on admission to the hospital, and there have been numerous examples where an overly aggressive treatment plan has been created by a hospitalist who is meeting a patient for the first time. One additional challenge for specialized hospital physicians is the lack of an established relationship with a critically ill patient and his or her family members. Recently, a hospitalist, entering a patient's room to meet with a family for the first time, notified the family that the patient's primary-care physician would not be coming to call on the patient. From that moment forward, the family and patient referred to the hospitalist as the "surprise doctor" or "Dr. Surprise."

Beyond the traditional acute hospital care setting, some physicians have further differentiated into developing the unique specialty of critical-care medicine, and they are known as "intensivists." Generally caring for the sickest of patients in the intensive care units of hospitals, these providers remain in very short supply and have been designated as an essential resource by some organizations that measure and report hospital quality and safety. One such organization, the Leapfrog Group, founded in 2000, is a nonprofit watchdog group whose focus is on improving the quality and safety of care being delivered in American hospitals to reduce unnecessary procedures, medical errors, and fraud.[31] As part of their work, the Leapfrog Group measures quality and safety using hospital surveys. The group delivers a performance grade for institutions that complete the survey, and nearly two thousand hospitals completed the

---

31 Leapfrog Hospital Safety Grade, accessed May 12, 2017, http://www.hospitalsafetygrade.org/about-us/about-the-leapfrog-group.

survey process in 2016.[32] One area of focus for Leapfrog has been in promoting the benefits of having specialty-trained intensivists in higher-performing hospitals, linking the presence of these physicians with a 30 percent reduction in hospital mortality and a 40 percent reduction in intensive care unit mortality in sites where intensivists are deployed.[33]

The final group of primary-care physicians to have evolved from the new model of care is a specialized group of practitioners who deal exclusively with the chronic care needs of individuals who reside in long–term care and post–acute care facilities. This emerging group, known as "SNFists" (caring for patients residing in "skilled nursing facilities"), have developed unique skills that enhance care for predominantly chronically ill and older patients confined in a long-term care site. When discharged from the hospital, elderly patients frequently have unresolved medical issues that require care outside the home, such as malnutrition, deconditioning weakness, and newly acquired conditions arising directly from their hospitalization that may include both physical and behavioral health components. The hope for this newest subset of clinicians is that they can oversee more coordinated care strategies for the people who are recovering from a hospitalization, generating lower costs of care while implementing better longitudinal care plans that will assist patients to more completely recapture their previous functional status and return home, where lower-intensity home services can be more appropriately delivered. Another major improvement expected from SNFist care is to create improved communication channels between clinical teams practicing in traditional ambulatory settings and care teams practicing within a hospital setting. This enhanced ability to pass along vital information between two apparently disparate groups will also assist patients and families as they try to piece together a comprehensive view of what transpired during a care experience and help set the expectations of what is likely to follow.

---

32 The Leapfrog Group website, accessed March 13, 2017, http://www.leapfroggroup.org/sites/default/files/Files/IPS%20Fact%20Sheet.pdf..

33 P. J. Pronovost, T. Young, T. Dorman, K. Robinson, and D. C. Angus, "Association between ICU Physician Staffing and Outcomes: A Systematic Review," *Critical Care Medicine* 27 (1999): A43.

A host of nontraditional health-care providers have also stepped in to fill a void recognized in traditional care approaches, with some demonstrating greater connectivity with existing systems of care and others that appear to be providing services that are best described as "one-offs" or "stand-alone" services. These new entrants, largely paid through retail out-of-pocket contributions from people who seek those relatively low-acuity health services, provide service convenience as the primary driver for health-care consumers. Many people have turned to these nontraditional providers mainly due to their close geographic location to home, which helps satisfy the consumer's demand for more timely access. Other reasons mentioned by health-care consumers for supplementing or replacing conventional services with retail providers is the manner with which retail service providers better understand the values-driven needs of a consumer, such as reduction in the administrative "hassle factor" during each encounter, reduction in wait times, assistance with completion of insurance paper work, and reduction in the work of the consumer to help with keeping a medical office record up to date.

An additional factor frequently cited by health-care consumers is that since they purchase health-care services as a commodity, price reigns supreme. There is a lengthy list of relatively uncomplicated clinical conditions that can be treated at retail pharmacy outlets, big-box stores with simplified medical clinics, and even stand-alone sites supported by health systems themselves. It is not unusual for a retail health clinic to provide a list of services and the exact cost for providing those services, the simplicity of which has been lacking in traditional health-care delivery sites. Many health systems have taken a stand to compete with retail outlets for access, but despite having physicians with office hours on Saturdays, Sundays, and evenings during the week, competition is stiff from retail, since they can provide significant pricing advantages for the well-defined conditions that are most often evaluated.

The second great financial disadvantage for health system office practices is that they are frequently called upon to care for an expanded array of clinical conditions, making the care experiences quite unpredictable with respect to consumer time demands. In a recent study published by Dr. Andrew Sussman in the *American Journal of Managed Care*, a pharmacy-based retail clinic was found to be less expensive in annual total costs of care with fewer visits to the emergency department when compared to conventional medical sites of service.[34] In addition to lower total costs of care, retail clinics have been shown to have superior-quality outcomes for commonly occurring medical conditions such as ear infections, sore throat, and urinary tract infection when compared to care delivered at traditional health system ambulatory care settings and in emergency departments.[35] The retail health clinics' share of the market has been steadily expanding. Commercial pharmacy sites operated nearly two thousand clinic sites that provided 10.8 million patient visits in 2014. In a retrospective review provided by Rand Health, the growth of retail clinic visits quadrupled between 2007 and 2009,[36] although the overall percentage of ambulatory visits was still dwarfed by traditional sites of care.

Aside from the emerging retail markets mentioned above, several virtual health-care sites have demonstrated promise for American health-care consumers as they attempt to find care advice at lower cost and greater convenience. Perhaps no communication channel has been used more by consumers than the World Wide Web, which has provided fingertip access to consumers seeking medical advice or support through open-access communication with other consumers. Several instant-access health-care information sites have been established by groups such as "big data" information technology sites, commercial health insurance vendors, holistic care resources, and employer-based health plans. Virtuwell from HealthPartners provides online appointments with certified nurse practitioners for a fixed price of forty-five dollars per online "visit" with a 100 percent service guarantee and the ability to have prescriptions delivered directly to the person's local pharmacy.[37] Enhancing

34 A. Sussman et al., "Retail Clinic Utilization Associated with Lower Total Costs of Care," *American Journal of Managed Care* (April 2013): e148–e157, accessed March 13, 2017.

35 W. H. Shrank et al., "Quality of Care at Retail Clinics for 3 Common Conditions," *American Journal of Managed Care* 20, no. 10 (2014): 794–801.

36 M. Mehrotra and J. Lave, "Visits to Retail Clinics Grew Fourfold from 2007 to 2009, although Their Share of Overall Outpatient Visits Remains Small," *Health Affairs* 31, no. 9 (2012): 2123–2129.

37 Virtuwell by Health Partners, "Welcome to Virtuwell, Your 24/7 Online Clinic," accessed May 12, 2017, https://www.virtuwell.com/.

convenience even further, Virtuwell files insurance claims on behalf of the patient and treats sixty of the most common medical conditions, receiving a 98 percent customer satisfaction rating.

Health systems and employers have also entered the retail sector to promote and maintain their prowess to provide comprehensive and integrated health-care services. Models of care delivery that embrace Internet and non-traditional care sites have also sprung forth as a variety of expanded services that include relaxation techniques, acupressure and acupuncture, massage, wellness, weight loss, and exercise programs have provided opportunities for health systems to demonstrate value as an integrator of services most needed by health-care consumers. Having made significant investments in information-technology infrastructure as part of the ascent of the electronic medical record, integrated health-care delivery systems are making efforts to use this innovative technology to provide direct-to-consumer applications and products. Beginning with providing access to a patient's own electronic medical record using patient information portals with virtual access to the medical record and thumb drives that can provide health information for patients to take with them to other health systems for care when on vacation or when traveling for business, access to the electronic medical record has become much more sophisticated in response to patient preferences.

As care consumers began to appreciate the value of having an accurate medical record with them at all times and at all locations, they also began demanding access to traditional health-care providers from the comforts of home. Secure websites with HIPAA-protected medical information replaced a patient's need to phone the physician's office to inquire about test results or to ask for medical advice. Dialogue now results when patients asynchronously ask medical questions and physicians respond to those inquiries after office hours. A primary-care physician colleague who has embraced the evolution of the electronic medical record confided that he spends from two to three hours each night answering medical queries from his patients, and each response is given free of charge, since there exists no reimbursement methodology for providing these answers. Unlike other professions where payment for time invested is part of the professional billing model, health care has long viewed the responsibility of answering questions posed by their patients as just a routine part of the services they provide to their patients. Unlike billing for units of time spent on telephone conversations as attorneys do, many physicians freely give their time to answer health queries after office hours, giving way to even greater access to those they serve through asynchronous dialogue through electronic patient portals.

A recent adjustment is the service arrangement that comes in the form of telemedicine, in which a patient can more synchronously access health services using a computer interface. Physicians use traditional examination tools that have been modified for application to the computer visit, and a charge for the consultation is made to the patient, typically paid by most insurance companies. Initially envisioned as a means of securing better access to physicians where services are in short supply, such as dermatology, where "a picture is worth a thousand words," the telemedicine service industry has virtually exploded over the past two decades. New care applications, such as virtual intensive care unit monitoring, can be provided by a centralized group of critical-care physicians who are in constant communication with the nurses who are present at a patient's bedside.[38] Further augmenting these services, computerized robots are being deployed at some sites where patients can be visited in their rooms in the hospital, with the robots transmitting observational data back to remote physicians.[39] Some advanced medical clinics, such as the Mayo Clinic in Rochester, Minnesota, have used telemedicine to support their Mayo Clinic Care Network, a group of predominantly rural and frontier hospitals where consultations with Mayo specialist physicians can be provided using a computer interface and electronic diagnostic tools that the

---

38 S. Kumar, S. Merchant, and R. Reynolds, "Tele-ICU: Efficacy and Cost-Effectiveness of Remotely Managing Critical Care," *Perspectives in Health Information Management* (Spring 2013), AHIMA Foundation, accessed March 14, 2017.

39 M. Becevic et al., "Robotic Telepresence in a Medical Intensive Care Unit—Clinicians' Perspectives," *Perspectives in Health Information Management* (Summer 2015), AHIMA Foundation, accessed March 4, 2017.

patient can use to provide the data needed to help the specialist formulate a diagnosis from hundreds of miles away.[40]

The final way in which the new health-care team is being reformatted is tied to health-care information that can be provided by care consumers directly back to clinician hubs from "biowearables" that transmit peripheral monitoring data such as heart rate, body temperature, electrocardiographic displays, and even skin salt content.[41] These devices, best described as mini-computers using wearable sensors, are showing great promise to assist health-care consumers by transmitting concurrent medical information regarding medical conditions that are being monitored remotely, thus promoting self-care and convenience.

Dr. Daniel Kraft, a Harvard-trained internist-pediatrician who completed his training in cancer medicine at Stanford University, founded IntelliMedicine, which focuses on integrated personalized medicine.[42] Kraft, with whom I shared a speaking engagement at the Wharton School of Business at the University of Pennsylvania, has been known to wear numerous remote medical monitoring devices to demonstrate the prowess of "biowearables" in making diagnoses and providing more convenient access to health-care services.[43] As he brings to life his personal tale of the evolving "electronic age" approach to personalized management of a small lump found on his neck, he is able to walk an audience through the telemedicine exercise from the initial diagnosis made via cell-phone camera images sent to a remote dermatologist; to online scheduling of necessary preoperative screening tests; to online scheduling of a minor surgical procedure in an ear, nose, and throat doctor's office to excise the lump; and finally to completing his care experience as he received a final diagnosis from

40 "Telehealth: When Technology Meets Health Care," Mayo Clinic Healthy Lifestyle website, last modified May 24, 2014, accessed March 14, 2017, http://www.mayoclinic.org/healthy-lifestyle/consumer-health/in-depth/telehealth/art-20044878.

41 J. Heikenfeld, "Sweat Sensors Will Change How Wearables Track Your Health," *IEEE Spectrum*, October 22, 2014, accessed May 12, 2017, http://spectrum.ieee.org/biomedical/diagnostics/sweat-sensors-will-change-how-wearables-track-your-health.

42 Speakers on Healthcare, "The Heartbeat of the Platform," accessed March 14, 2017, http://www.speakersonhealthcare.com/speakers/Daniel_Kraft_MD.php.

43 Wharton School of Business, MBA Student-Led Conference, Philadelphia, Pennsylvania, April 2014.

an online anatomic pathologist. The entire in-person time spent was in the very brief encounter when the surgeon performed the actual minor excisional procedure. All other parts of the process, from initial diagnosis to final treatment, were carried out from the comfort of his home using his personal cellular devices.

The new models of care delivery that are still evolving as we approach the end of the second decade of the twenty-first century have left providers and consumers challenged by the many ways that a care consumer may secure access to health-care services. No longer is there a singular relationship between one individual consuming health care and one individual delivering that care. We now have "medical homes" where multiple services within a health system can be organized, and even "medical neighborhoods" where services from several interdependent health-care provider businesses come together. Multiple funding schemes have been proposed to harness this expanding set of services that are loosely organized within the new care system, but in the end, the health-care experience still centers on a single individual who is accessing the care needed to remain healthy or to treat injury and illness. Writing in the *Journal of the American Medical Association*, Lipstein and Kellerman identify several key recommendations that are necessary requirements as we define the workforce needed in the twenty-first-century health-care system.[44] They believe that four key issues need to be addressed in workforce development:

- ***Health professionals to steward health and health care.*** The authors believe that greater focus on the primary and preventive care needs of individuals can not only preserve health status, but do so at much lower costs than allowing diseases to develop and progress toward end-stage conditions. When conditions are allowed to progress, greater resources are needed to fully diagnose their extent and spread, and more expensive therapies are frequently required.
- ***Telehealth.*** With the hope that individuals can receive modern health care without having to travel long distances, the authors believe that

---

44 S. H. Lipstein and A. L. Kellerman, "Workforce for 21st-Century Health and Health Care," *Journal of the American Medical Association* 316, no. 16 (2016): 1665–1666.

health-care consumers can demand to be evaluated and treated at home at a lower overall cost when access to remote specialized providers can be secured. Instead of requiring consumers to travel long distances to see these providers in person, telemedicine services can minimize patient inconvenience, decrease lost productivity from time spent traveling, reduce costs associated with travel to specialized providers, and result in better health outcomes, as more accurate diagnoses are given when consumers have access to specialized providers that are not available in most local communities.

- **Clinicians to manage chronic, often co-occurring conditions.** With multiple health conditions simultaneously affecting individuals, the workforce of the future will need to be a diverse, interdisciplinary team composed of traditional care providers engaged with many other types of service providers. This integrated and interdependent team can assist in establishing more comprehensive treatment plans that address issues such as a person's nutritional status, outlining substance abuse and behavioral health strategies, and bringing forth rehabilitative medicine services. As a former health-system CEO informed me, the best system is one that can define and deliver the needed services, delivered by the right person, for the right reasons, and at just the right time.

- **Caregivers at the end of life.** The authors call for greater emphasis on deployment of additional resources for palliative and hospice care to help patients who are approaching the end of their lives. Compassionate care delivery using models that address the values-driven needs of people who are facing difficult care decisions will become paramount. The degree of intensity expected in services delivered and how far to pursue the vast array of health services that are available to assure the most appropriate services will go a long way toward helping create sensitive and patient-directed approaches to care delivery. Many pilots are underway to help sponsor better communication with individuals approaching the end of life, and improved structures that support the wishes of these patients are being evaluated, such as the Age-Friendly

Health System project jointly sponsored by the John A. Hartford Foundation and the Institute for Health Care Improvement.[45]

The impact from redesign of these new teams and services reflects a recognition that there are changing requirements for the use of any health-care delivery system. Evolving structures must organically emerge with new and better solutions provided to meet the needs of today's consumers, but they must do so without sacrificing the historic and personal bond that has connected the health-care consumer and health-care provider for hundreds of years. Recognizing that the health-care experience is still a very human endeavor, new delivery strategies will need to fully embrace the many strengths realized from delivering the optimal care in the most caring fashion. As new systems of care are being constructed, attention must be paid to how evolving delivery networks can exploit the humanistic best from the past while still promoting new breakthroughs in technology. The health-care delivery team of the future, working with a more activated group of health-care consumers, will intentionally design these new systems and match them with new models for care funding being proposed through federal and state health policies. This threading of a needle to produce a system of care that works for all Americans will not emerge as an isolated and disjointed structure; instead, it will focus on solutions that maintain the very personal relationship between care consumers and care providers needed to maintain the human bond that has always been at the heart of health care.

---

45 The John A. Hartford Foundation, "Age-Friendly Health Systems," accessed May 12, 2017, http://www.johnahartford.org/grants-strategy/current-strategies/age-friendly-hospitals/.

Key Points to Master From Chapter 4

- The new health delivery system paradigm calls for provision of medical services that are of highest quality and safety at a lower cost (high value) by aligning and integrating treatment teams and continuum partners (network development), leveraging these capabilities to drive differentiation and viability in the changing healthcare environment (enhanced financial outcomes).

- Multiple causes for provider burnout: greater complexity and knowledge needed to master, physician employment with increasing time pressures creating a focus on the health care "transactions" and "productivity rewards", decreased autonomy, depersonalization of the provider-patient bond, use of electronic health records that distract some clinicians from their patients, public reporting of quality and safety data.

- With shrinking physician numbers, personnel are stepping up to deliver and extend care sites of service, ranging from informal assistants working under direct supervision to more autonomous physician assistants and nurse practitioners.

- New physician roles are emerging, including "hospitalists" who care for hospitalized patients, "intensivists" who care for the sickest patients in the intensive care units, "SNFists" who provide care in nursing homes, and "office-based primary care physicians" who do not see hospitalized patients.

- Expanded retail provider roles include: pharmacists and nurses working in retail clinic settings owned by pharmacy companies and Big Box stores, online blogs and advice, "virtual visits" such as telemedicine, and the use of "biowearables" to better connect health care consumers with the expanded set of care providers.

- Workforce development will need to focus on the following:
  - Health professionals will always be needed to steward health and the health care experience; coordinating their roles is essential.

o   Telehealth will continue to provide greater access to asynchronous care.
o   Chronic and co-occurring conditions will require specialized clinicians.
o   As people live longer with greater illness burden, specialized providers to assist people with advanced care directives and end-of-life decision-making will be needed to meet person-centered values being expressed.

Five

THE EMERGING HEALTH-CARE CONSUMER

N ot only has the provider context changed over that past half century, but the people consuming care have also redefined themselves. No longer passive participants in the health-care delivery dance, consumers now are described as "activated" and "engaged" in their effort to gain greater value from the health-care delivery system.[46] A new cottage industry that supports "patient and family engagement" has also sprung up, with the newly minted term "patient advocates" being charged with becoming the "social designers of the care experience."[47,48] What has this done to the relationship between health-care providers and health-care consumers? To understand where we are currently and where the future is leading us, a better understanding of how we arrived at this moment is necessary.

When "old Doc Henslin" approached my mother and me about his plan to remove my tonsils in his office, he was acting with the kind paternal benevolence of the 1950s and 1960s. Knowing that my mother had no medical

---

46 J. Hibbard and J. Greene, "What the Evidence Shows about Patient Activation: Better Health Outcomes and Care Experiences; Fewer Data on Costs," *Health Affairs* 32, no. 2 (2013): 207–214.

47 "The Assertive Patient: Speaking Up When You Are Dissatisfied with a Health Care Experience," accessed May 15, 2017, http://www.assertivepatient.org/patient-advocate.html.

48 Patient Advocate Foundation, "Solving Insurance and Healthcare Access Problems," accessed May 15, 2017, http://patientadvocate.org/.

training or experience, he accepted his social role as transcendent caregiver and provided his best advice based on his personal medical experience and training. I'm certain that it must have been shocking to him when my mother decided that she was not going to bring me to the office for such a procedure, not for medical reasons but rather for financial reasons. My father, a very hardworking parts manager at a local Ford dealership, was barely making enough to support a family of four, independent of any medical issues that might rear their ugly heads. My mother was not acting out as a disgruntled relative, but was merely hoping that her faith in God would bring me through a bout of severe tonsillitis without having to undergo an expensive procedure. In the end—and not because of her medical insight, my mother proved to be prescient—my tonsils lived to see another day.

Much has changed since those days of benevolent paternalism, and a great deal is directly tied to people finding their own competency to act on information that is now becoming more readily available. This newfound position of being a more informed health-care consumer came from a struggle wrought with starts and stops, with medical information sometimes being passed on without appropriate context, leading to many difficult conversations between patients and physicians mired in past relationships that were based on the historic social compact between the two groups. As information began to be published in lay press resources, changes in how medical recommendations were transmitted and received were initially very poorly developed, with grandmotherly advice embedded in general writings such as *The World Book Encyclopedia*[49] and *McCall's Magazine*.[50]

When told that I had an inguinal hernia that had been found during a routine prefootball sports physical, I quickly turned to the best reference we had in the house, my trusted 1957 set of *The World Book* with its red-and-blue spine inscribed with gold letters and numbers. Pulling volume 8 (letter H), I explored the information a physician would use to diagnose a "hernia" and reviewed the many options for how the condition should be treated. Remembering back to the days when my mother had advised us not to have

---

49 *The World Book Encyclopedia* (Chicago: Simon & Schuster, 1957).
50 *McCall's Magazine: The First Magazine for Women* (McCall Corporation, last published 2002).

surgical interventions, I was hoping to find reassurance that my condition could just be safely monitored without any significant consequence. I was shocked to find that if such a hernia were to strangulate, gangrene could set in, and a person with such a painful complication could die due to rupture of the entrapped bowel or due to widespread infection that would result. Perhaps I missed the fine details of the *World Book* discussion, but I clearly remember that the subject was far too complicated for me to understand as a twelve-year-old footballer, and I laid the topic aside and happily trotted out to the practice field to begin my football career without incident. Just as with the tonsillectomy, the hernia continued without incident over the course of my life, reinforcing the lesson that not all things diagnosed necessarily needed to be treated. I also learned that reading about medical conditions without context could send shivers up the spine of an impressionable young boy.

The shift away from medical paternalism began in the 1970s and 1980s as a sense of empowered decision-making swept across American consumers in many other fields. Purchasing decisions for products ranging from blenders to automobiles were made easier with information provided by *Consumer Reports*,[51] "advising Americans since 1936." Health-care consumption, however, has always been a bit different, and when consumers began a crusade to promote their participation in more informed health-care decisions, it was initially quite challenging for providers who were still stuck in the philosophy that they would bear the sole responsibility to "do things *to* their patients." Health-care consumers began viewing encounters with their providers as needing to be more inclusive of their preferences, and physicians either resisted this new approach to the social compact or embraced the change.

Many enlightened practitioners began considering the values of a patient and family as they adopted a new way of doing business, shifting to a new philosophy of "doing things *for* a patient." Discussions between providers and consumers began to embrace the concerns for the whole person, and a great deal of literature was beginning to be published about how providers

51 *Consumer Reports*, published by Consumers Union, accessed March 29, 2017, http://consumersunion.org/.

and consumers might work together to design better patient care experiences.[52] Instead of just assuming a patient's need for a specific intervention that was hand-selected by the provider, discussions began to yield joint decisions crafted by the values reflected by both the person providing care and the person receiving care. This "values-driven decision-making" served as a breakthrough in establishing a more mature relationship between the two parties that further changed the social compact between them. Patients were now seen as more than just childlike individuals who needed the wisdom and guidance of a learned physician, and a spirit of creating an effective shared experience became a cornerstone of the new relationship.

As consumerism progressed through the end of the twentieth century, organized groups promoting patient engagement arrived on the scene, advocating for greater inclusion of patients around the medical decision-making table.[53,54] These groups began reframing the relationship once again, shifting from the more passive "doing things *for* my patients" to a more active approach of "doing things *with* patients," where people consuming care were demanding to be included in any decision about their care. By becoming more actively engaged, "patients" became "health-care consumers" and began to provide meaningful assistance to health-care provider teams in a successful approach that formulated more comprehensive person-focused treatment plans.

Beginning with the 2001 publication *Crossing the Quality Chasm* from the Institute of Medicine, which outlined the Six Aims needed to improve the twenty-first-century health-care system,[55] high-value care was challenged to become more patient-centered at its core. This conclusion had been drawn from years of study of improved patient outcomes that arose from greater

52 M. D. Naylor and W. D. Novelli, "Care Culture and Decision-Making," *National Academy of Medicine*, accessed May 15, 2017, https://nam.edu/programs/value-science-driven-health-care/care-culture-and-decision-making/.

53 J. Sammer, "Promoting Health Care Consumerism: A Multifaceted Approach," *Society for Human Resource Management*, November 3, 2011, accessed May 15, 2017, https://www.shrm.org/ResourcesAndTools/hr-topics/benefits/Pages/Consumerism.aspx.

54 Agency for Healthcare Research and Quality, accessed May 15, 2017, https://www.ahrq.gov/patients-consumers/index.html.

55 W. C. Richardson, chairman, Committee on Quality of Health Care in America, *Crossing the Quality Chasm* (Washington, DC: National Academy Press, 2001).

degrees of patient involvement in developing care plans. Giving patients more autonomy and self-control has been associated with many benefits, and some researchers have identified two key steps that help reinforce a provider's commitment to every health-care consumer to achieve such patient-centeredness: build a meaningful role for patients and families into every care experience and customize patient care to stimulate patients to develop mastery of their own health-promotion activities.[56]

From a publication in late 2015,[57] strategies and tactics that have been put in place since the beginning of the patient-and-family engagement movement include enhancing the ways in which health information can be better transmitted and understood (health literacy), engagement strategies needed during hospitalization, encouraging patients and families to more actively design care experiences that will result in better health outcomes, partnering with health system leadership and governance, reducing health-care disparities, and improving the process for generating health-care decisions that can be shared by provider and consumer. The publication cites the many ways in which health-care processes can be improved by more deeply engaging patients and families, with beneficial results seen in quality[58] and patient safety,[59] cost efficiency,[60] and provider[61] and patient satisfaction. As patients and their families become

---

56 J. Hibbard and J. Greene, "Engaged Patients Translate to Better Outcomes and Costs," *The Health Care Blog*, February 10, 2013, accessed March 29, 2017, http://thehealthcareblog.com/blog/2013/02/10/engaged-patients-translate-to-better-outcomes-and-costs/.

57 *Patient and Family Engagement Resource Compendium* (Chicago: Health Research & Educational Trust, December 2015), accessed March 29, 2017, www.hpoe.org.

58 S. N. Weingart et al., "Hospitalized Patients' Participation and Its Impact on Quality of Care and Patient Safety," *International Journal for Quality in Health Care* 23:269–77, accessed March 29, 2017, http://intqhc.oxfordjournals.org/content/23/3/269.

59 M. Stewart "The Impact of Patient-Centered Care on Outcomes," *Journal of Family Practice* 49, no. 9 (2000): 796–804, accessed March 29, 2017, http://www.mdedge.com/jfponline/article/60893/impact-patient-centered-care-outcomes.

60 K. D. Bertakis and R. Azari, "Patient-Centered Care Is Associated with Decreased Health Care Utilization," *Journal of the American Board of Family Medicine* 24, no. 3 (2011): 229–39, accessed March 29, 2017, http://www.jabfm.org/content/24/3/229.full.pdf+html.

61 P. Rosen et al., "Family-Centered Multidisciplinary Rounds Enhance the Team Approach in Pediatrics," *Pediatrics* 123, no.4 (2009): e603–e608, www.pediatrics.org/cgi/content/ full/123/4/e603.

more involved in their own episodes of care as activated participants, health-care delivery systems can better customize the care delivery spaces as places of healing and improving care experiences that lead directly to better health outcomes.[62] "Patient activation" implies that a patient's knowledge, skills, and abilities enhance the intrinsic management of that person's health care, while "patient engagement" combines patient activation approaches with efforts to promote positive patient behaviors that reinforce a new approach to care delivery.[63] This new paradigm, years in the making, promotes shared decision-making rather than simply accepting the traditional approach of assessing the inherent medical complexity of care delivery systems as a barrier that only a trained health professional could understand to orchestrate diagnostic and therapeutic decisions. This approach takes time, given the need for a thorough review of each patient's condition, a review of the many therapeutic options, and an assessment of the benefits and risk of each and how these fit with the patient's individual preferences.

One such example of taking the time needed to understand a patient and family's unique preferences comes from my previous medical practice as a nephrologist, when a sweet ninety-eight-year-old great-grandmother was referred to me to initiate dialysis treatments for her kidney failure. Following a long discussion with this kindly woman and her family, it became clear that this very clear-thinking patient had little prior understanding of what had been proposed for her by her primary-care doctor. As we discussed the options for her treatment, she became most interested when I suggested that she also had an option to receive no dialysis at all, but to approach her clinical condition with very conservative goals that would focus on keeping her comfortable as her kidney disease progressed. She became a great advocate for herself at this point, asking several questions about the final phases of end-stage kidney disease and whether she would experience any pain or suffering should she make the decision not to proceed with more aggressive treatment. Her children,

---

62 M. Joshi et al., *Leading Health Care Transformation: A Primer for Clinical Leaders* (Boca Raton, FL: CRC Press, 2016).

63 "Patient Engagement," Health Policy Brief, *Health Affairs*, February 14, 2013, accessed March 29, 2017, http://healthaffairs.org/healthpolicybriefs/brief_pdfs/healthpolicybrief_86.pdf.

who had suggested the referral to me for dialysis out of love for their mother, began to better understand their mother's preferences for various treatment interventions, and they began framing clinical decisions in terms of the values of their mother. In the end, this wonderful mother, grandmother, and great-grandmother opted to receive supportive care only, deferring any plan for dialysis treatments. She provided me a lasting lesson in the importance of taking the time to listen from the heart, engaging on a very human level and feeling comfortable with placing the final decision in the hands of the person who was most invested in the decisions being made, the patient herself.

In terms of shared decision-making, several principles can be illustrated from this joint care plan formulation. First, we both knew that we needed to make a decision; her clinical condition was progressing, and without an active decision being made, we were in fact making a decision. Second, the medical evidence describing the condition at hand and its potential treatment options needed to be explained in such a way that a person without medical training could meaningfully engage in active decision-making. Finally, questions needed to be asked of the patient to allow her to express her values and preferences for care. From there, the options for therapy could be compared, and the patient then had the opportunity to exercise her right to participate in the creation of her personalized treatment plan. These steps mirror the approach offered by Bisognano and Goodman in their landmark article written in 2013 that describes the respectful conversations needed to be held with patients and families as the person actively makes choices about proceeding with technically complex health-care interventions made near the end of his or her life.[64]

When several provider treatment preferences markedly differ, or when provider preferences clash with those of a patient and a family, great confusion as to how to proceed is often seen. This can arise when multiple approaches with minor differences in treatment effect are considered simultaneously. As

---

64 M. Bisognano and E. Goodman, "Engaging Patients and Their Loved Ones in the Ultimate Conversation," *Health Affairs* 32, no. 2 (2013): 203–206, accessed March 29, 2017, http://content.healthaffairs.org/content/32/2/203.full.

an example from a recent survey published in 2014,[65] it is clear that specialty physicians representing surgical and radiation therapy specialties continue to reflect a difference of opinion regarding how best to treat prostate cancer. The conclusion of the study suggested that patients may be receiving biased information based on the specialty provider who renders that guidance, and that if truly informed consent were to be provided to patients hoping to participate in shared decision-making, those individuals would need to consult with radiation-therapy doctors to discuss the risks and benefits of radiation treatment of prostate cancer while also conferring with a urologist to better comprehend the risks and benefits of more invasive surgical therapy. The surprising thing about the study was not just that differences of opinion exist among very knowledgeable specialists, but that the debate between those favoring radiation treatment and those recommending surgical treatment has continued for so many years without clear resolution of treatment advantage. How, then, should a new-age health-care consumer come to an independent decision about the best care for oneself when the experts cannot even come to an agreement?

People seeking assistance in making informed care decisions are not expecting perfection but rather just some degree of clarity that will come when all parties involved in such important decisions have an opportunity to put forth their well-researched impressions for how to proceed. Health-care consumers are only asking to have their values considered and to hold a seat at the table when such important decisions are being made. Further, today's health-care consumers want to feel as if they have a voice that can help providers create more individualized health-care treatment plans, and they also want to contribute to a more systematic improvement in health system design that recognizes patient-centered approaches to care delivery. This recent trend of involving patients and families in health-care process redesign has led to breakthrough innovations, since these new members of the design team come to an improvement project without the narrow thinking that has limited health-care

---

65 S. P. Kim et al., "Specialty Bias in Treatment Recommendations and Quality of Life among Radiation Oncologists and Urologists for Localized Prostate Cancer," *Prostate Cancer and Prostatic Diseases* 17 (June 2014): 163–169.

professionals who look through the more traditional lens of inertia. Providers tend to see work processes the way they have always been rather than looking at a host of untested possibilities that are frequently identified by consumers of those care processes.

From a previous example of "seeing through a patient's eyes," the IDEO Corporation was able to demonstrate the new "voice of the customer" approach by providing fresh construction design ideas for a cardiovascular center simply because they came to the project without any idea of what the ultimate project *should* look like, focusing instead on the goal of including patient preferences and perspectives in the design.[66] These "next level" solutions came to life through an ideation process that focused on safety, clarity, information exchange, and customer mapping that helped embed patient preferences into the design of a new heart center. The design reflected how a facility could best be used by patients and families, reinforcing how innovative solutions could lead to a facility that not only exceeded the community's expectations, but also resulted in better and safer care practices.

In practical terms, then, how does one create an environment in which health-care providers and health-care consumers can come together to realize the impact seen when they clearly express their preferences? What does this mean to twenty-first-century health care, and what benefits will arise from such deep engagement of activated participants? What are the initial steps that providers need to take to recognize the importance of consumer input into the next generation of health-care strategies that better recognize the preferences of those who are using the health-care system? Evidence exists that demonstrates the ways that designing and deploying a new set of strategies helps create a more respectful and more effective environment that incorporates patient preferences. Following a review of those suggestions for designing experiences that invite consumer design, examples can illustrate where health-care delivery systems use these tactics to reimagine their health-care processes, bringing the delivery system more in line with several of the Institute of Medicine's Six Aims to make health care more predictably effective, efficient, and patient-centered.

---

66 P. A. Newbold and D. Stover-Hopkins, *Wake Up and Smell the Innovation: Stirring Up a Return on !magination* (Networlding Publishing, 2013).

Strategies for activating participants and promoting patient and family engagement can come at two levels, adapted from a model provided by Kristin Carman and associates at the American Institutes for Research. One strategy calls for promotion of a tactical approach to individual patient and family decision making, while the second approach calls for more active patient and family participation in health care process redesign.[67] From Carman's research, the definition of patient and family engagement as "patients, families, and their representatives, and health professionals working in active partnership at various levels across the health care system" is offered. This mental model recognizes the importance of such an evolutionary relationship as patients and families become more active, informed, and influential in decision-making. While some commonalities exist between the two levels of influence, it is important to understand each in greater detail:

- *Individualized patient and family engagement efforts.* Much of the benefit that arises from incorporating the voices of individual patients and families results from enhanced information flow between care-delivery teams and those who are consuming the care. This can typically be deployed best by providing ease of access to such clinical information through a variety of bidirectional communication conduits, the most powerful of which is the electronic health record. When providers seek information-technology solutions that engage patients and their loved ones into system design, enhanced methods can be used to collect, aggregate, and utilize information that is vital to a better understanding of how care processes are being recreated for "person-focused" delivery. By engaging patients and families in a meaningful two-way conversation about those strategies, patient preferences help guide the care plan in a more productive direction. At its most primitive, patients should have access to clinical notes and conclusions to help correct inaccuracies and allow these conclusions to be used in fruitful discussions about proposed next steps in

---

67 K. Carman et al., "Patient and Family Engagement: A Framework for Understanding the Elements and Developing Interventions and Policies," *Health Affairs* 32, no. 2 (2013): 223–231.

treatment planning, including preferences for diagnostic tools and interventions. As greater engagement is seen, patients can begin asynchronous conversations through electronic information portals that engage providers and consumers in a manner that more efficiently uses their time to ask and answer back. Having direct access to laboratory and radiology reports, patients can ask clarifying questions that can be answered after conventional work hours by clinicians, leading to a deeper understanding of the next steps needed to complete a diagnostic evaluation.

Another way in which direct input can be received from patients and families is though inpatient interdisciplinary rounding that engages all members of the treatment team to be present at one time to discuss the clinical context with a patient and family.[68,69] Having the opportunity to transparently communicate through person-focused dialogue not only helps patients and families feel more engaged, it is a very efficient way to make certain that thorough and accurate depictions of a treatment plan are clearly communicated by all members of the care team. Finally, some intentional efforts to promote more effective communication at the time of discharge can also help translate the discharge planning steps and prevent gaps in understanding of what the patient and family should do following discharge. Using an adult education method for effective information transfer, nursing staff provide information to a patient who then must "teach back" that same information to the discharge coordinator to make certain that it has been effectively communicated.[70] Citing the potential for confusion between provider and patient roles and the health

---

68 K. J. O'Leary, R. Buck, H. M. Fligiel, et al., "Structured Interdisciplinary Rounds in a Medical Teaching Unit: Improving Patient Safety," *The JAMA Network: JAMA Internal Medicine*, April 11, 2011.

69 K. J. O'Leary, N. L. Sehgal, G. Terrell, et al., "Interdisciplinary Teamwork in Hospitals: A Review and Practical Recommendations for Improvement," *Journal of Hospital Medicine* (2011), accessed May 15, 2017.

70 H. McFarland, M. Kirn, and A. Williams, *CAT Teach Back Method of Discharge Instructions* (Kansas City, MO: Children's Mercy Hospital).

outcomes that need to be measured to document clinical improvements directly related to better patient engagement, Epstein calls for even more patient-centered care, if for no other reason than a recognition that today's health-care consumers will grow to be more involved in leading their own care teams.[71]

The importance of comanagement that relies on both health-care consumers and care providers reveals a need to remember that these communication channels operate in both directions. When care providers use these channels to relay critical instructions to a care consumer, the care team then holds itself accountable to an outcome that has been agreed upon by both interested parties, and adherence to tactics outlined in a care plan can be documented in the medical record. A fellow resident-in-training at Iowa Lutheran Hospital encouraged a patient and family to discuss the importance of smoking cessation, as the patient was beginning to demonstrate early signs of significant lung disease associated with a long history of tobacco abuse. When the patient stated that he would not agree to adhere to such a recommendation, it provided the impetus for the young physician to hold a frank conversation with the family about helping the patient find a different doctor who might be more tolerant of the patient's cigarette smoking. In the previous days of benevolent paternalism, a care provider might otherwise feel compelled to continue forward with the patient, since adherence with recommendations was a problem owned unilaterally by the physician.

• *Patient and family roles in health-care process design and governance.* Several health-care organizations have experimented with patient representation at listening sessions to capture their responses to proposed strategic directions of that organization. It has become apparent only recently that health-care processes can be significantly improved through stronger engagement of patients and families during the design phase of new therapies, care processes, and facility

---

71 R. Epstein and R. Street, "The Values and Value of Patient-Centered Care," *Annals of Family Medicine* 9, no. 2 (2011): 100–103.

design. What had historically been a passive role of providing feedback on already established conclusions reached by health systems has shifted to a new role for patients and families serving as more meaningfully engaged advisors to and partners with health systems. From Newbold and Stover-Hopkins's work at Memorial Health System in South Bend, Indiana, deploying principles to stimulate more active patient involvement in designing systems and processes of care can be shown to bear fruit.[72] Not only can an organization prevent errors of commission resulting from construction planning without first seeking customer input, but also significant financial savings can be realized, as consumer coordination can help guide facility construction that promotes greater community loyalty.

An interesting design I once viewed related to construction of a new emergency department that was being planned. It demonstrated a beautiful waiting space with soft lounge chairs, a warm greeting and nursing triage area that provided privacy for sensitive conversations regarding clinical information, a private dictation and medical records area for physicians to work in comfortable privacy, private exam spaces with great lighting, and access to the latest in medical technology. However, one major design flaw was noted in the placement of an ear, nose, and throat (ENT) examination space for treatment of children with ear infections and nosebleeds. To move from the emergency department entrance to the ENT examination area, children would have had to walk past a major trauma room where people who had been injured in automobile accidents were being evaluated. Without consumer feedback regarding this plan design, children would have been exposed to patients with broken bones, bleeding arteries from severe lacerations, and screaming and crying patients and loved ones, all of which would surely have terrified an impressionable youngster with an earache!

---

72 Newbold and Stover-Hopkins, *Wake Up and Smell the Innovation.*

Beyond the design of care facilities for patient-centeredness, health-care consumers and their families have emerged as some of the best advisors for health-care process redesign. Having directly experienced the results from imprecise care process design, consumers can provide valuable input into needed changes in care practices without having the limitations of the initial bias found in so many care providers. The expression "but that's the way we've always done it" is all too frequently heard in conversations with providers regarding process change, but since patients and families have no historic bias for what "must be true," they can give candid feedback that brings out defects that might otherwise go unnoticed.

More advanced health systems are engaging patients and families as partners in helping promote higher degrees of quality and safety. I recently held a telephone conversation with Dr. David Pryor, a physician leader serving as the executive vice president for Ascension Health Alliance in St. Louis. He stated that his organization had made great strides in producing more predictable outcomes from their redesigned care practices, operating at levels as low as one defect in one hundred thousand patient encounters. While he stressed that much of the care improvement had occurred because of Ascension's engagement of patients in care redesign, he felt that there was still one remaining improvement step that could yield even greater benefit. Pryor cited the "last great frontier" of fully engaging patients and families at all levels of the organization's improvement efforts, aiming for a defect rate of one in a million encounters by taking this final leap of patient engagement. A full list of roles for patients and families can be found in Joshi's *Primer for Clinical Leaders* with a discussion on how best to partner with patients and families to achieve high reliability.[73] These roles include storytelling and education sessions, participation on quality and safety teams, reviewing patient materials, developing care coordination strategies, helping with facility design, improving

---

73 Joshi et al., *Leading Health Care Transformation*.

function of information technology patient portals, and serving as advisors to executive leadership and the board of directors.

Although barriers certainly can exist in finding ways to engage patients and families in redesigning current care experiences, most of these barriers are tied to a need to overcome the intrinsic inertia found in the current state of care delivery systems. When providers become open to the prospect of using patient and family feedback in a positive way, when health-care consumers overcome their natural fear and intimidation of dealing with such complex scientific findings, and when senior leaders overcome their disinclination to publicly air the defects that need to be improved, remarkable results can be realized that benefit all parties involved.

One final thought regarding the incorporation of patient and family feedback into health-care design is tied to the historically uncomfortable discussions related to how health-care consumers can express their values in making decisions as they approach the end of their lives, so-called advanced care planning decisions.[74,75] Perhaps no more sensitive discussion is held between a care provider and a care consumer than that of a person's intimate wishes regarding health-care strategies as the person approaches the end of life. Several organizations have spent countless years helping providers better understand the needs of an aging population to help plan for the inevitable, including the John A. Hartford Foundation's work on developing Age-Friendly Health Systems to promote implementation of evidence-based approaches to help health systems seek input from seniors and to help activate those same individuals to become leaders in expressing their own values-driven needs and decisions.[76] With a focus that goes well beyond helping aging individuals express their advanced care planning needs, the Hartford Foundation is attempting

74 Nous Foundation, "Advanced Care Planning Decisions," accessed May 15, 2017, https://www.acpdecisions.org/.

75 National Hospice and Palliative Care Organization, accessed May 15, 2017, https://www.nhpco.org/advance-care-planning.

76 "Age-Friendly Health Systems," John A. Hartford Foundation, accessed March 30, 2017, http://www.johnahartford.org/grants-strategy/current-strategies/age-friendly-hospitals/.

to promote person-sensitive approaches to care that will translate into better and safer care at lower costs that enhances the clinical outcomes as defined by the patients themselves. One other exemplar organization is Aging with Dignity from Tallahassee, Florida, whose Five Wishes campaign promotes a framework for sponsoring providers and consumers in their desire to hold advance care planning conversations.[77] By providing a series of five simple "wishes" that persons approaching the end of their life can express to their care teams, the organization hopes to bring forward a person's values that can be respected during this very vulnerable yet poorly understood time of life. The Five Wishes include discussions that explicitly clarify:

- The person I want to make care decisions for me when I can't.
- The kind of medical treatment I want and don't want.
- How comfortable I want to be.
- How I want people to treat me.
- What I want my loved ones to know.

Both approaches used by the Five Wishes group and the Hartford Foundation are grounded in the fundamental concept that health-care consumers deserve our respect and that all care providers should appreciate that each person should be entitled to express these preferences at such an important and vulnerable point in the health-care experience.

In work from David Schulke, principal for Health Quality Strategies LLC,[78] research has demonstrated that physicians are largely unprepared to hold conversations with their patients about issues at the end of one's life, and he calls for development of a "turnkey" training program that can be delivered to health systems that may not have the infrastructure to support the needed programs that focus on provider and consumer engagement. One such program currently in place was created by the Internal Medicine Residency Program at

---

77 Five Wishes, "Aging with Dignity," accessed March 30, 2017, www.agingwithdignity.org.
78 D. Schulke, Health Quality Strategies LLC, Annapolis, MD.

NorthShore University HealthSystems, based in Evanston, Illinois,[79] to help young physicians develop competencies around holding these delicate but very important conversations. Using a six-step approach to help providers prepare themselves for initiating patient and family meetings to better understand consumer wishes driven by their personal values, young doctors learn to plan for such discussions, frame probing questions that allow patients to personally express their desires, invite patients to actively participate in these discussions, promote acquisition of better communication skills to enhance such conversations, discuss goals of care, and hold empathic conversations that result in more intentional person-focused care strategies. The residents use a defined curriculum and video recordings that allow each trainee to observe their performance during simulated conversations to better create a comforting environment.

The important role of the health-care consumer has changed dramatically from the days of medical paternalism, and health-care providers are now relying on patients and families to help direct the care experiences that are becoming more effective and efficient as they focus on meeting another of the Institute of Medicine's Six Aims for twenty-first-century health care, that of delivering "patient-centered" health care. As the relationship between care provider and care consumer continues to mature over the next decade, it is anticipated that health-care "value" will begin to be more fully realized as the previously uninvited care consumer becomes the guest of honor at the health-care table.

---

79 NorthShore University HealthSystem Internal Medicine Residency Program, Evanston, IL, accessed March 31, 2017, http://www.northshore.org/academics/academic-programs/residency-programs/internal-medicine/..

Key Points to Master From Chapter 5

- "Benevolent paternalism" has been largely replaced by a new era of "health care consumerism" that shifted the focus from a provider being the final authority on all decisions to a more mature provider-consumer relationship that better focused on working together toward a comprehensive approach to care experiences.
- "Patient activation" implies that a patient's knowledge, skills, and abilities enhance the intrinsic management of a person's health care, while "patient engagement" combines patient activation with efforts to promote positive patient behaviors that reinforce a more holistic approach to care delivery plans.
- Two levels of patient and family engagement exist:
  o Individualized patient and family engagement efforts: securing enhanced information flow between care delivery teams and consumers of care.
  o Patient and family roles in health care process design and governance: redesigning care processes with the key input of consumers of care.
- The Five Wishes® campaign asks health care providers and consumers to address five essential questions when planning end-of-life care planning decisions.
- From the work of David Schulke and NorthShore University HealthSystem, six steps to train new physicians are outlined, with outstanding results demonstrating that skills to incorporate patient preferences can be incorporated into comprehensive approaches to care planning.

Six

CARE COORDINATION SYSTEMS—
REDUCING THE COST OF CARE

Two very simple parameters generally define the overall cost of American health care: the number of services used by American consumers and the cost per unit of service provided. Several mitigating factors will also be reviewed in this chapter, but for the purposes of the discussion of total cost of care, these two factors will be recognized as the most important drivers of the spiraling cost of health care. These cost determinants are also the most important components that have been proffered in a variety of health-care legislation proposals over the past century. Whether the discussion centers on vital cost elements such as variation in prescription of care services, the costs related to provision of low-quality services, or whether insurance rates are set reasonably to promote certain services that will lead to a reduction in the overall cost of care, the simple fact remains that the two key determinants of cost are the number of services being provided and the cost for each of these services.

The United States spends more than any other industrialized nation on health-care service delivery, and elevating care delivery to a status of a "medical-care industrial complex" implies that health care as an industry has become too big to fail given its impact on the nation's gross domestic product tied directly to provision of those services.[80,81,82] The most important question that has been recently asked as health-care legislation continues to be proposed, debated, passed, and then repealed is whether the services that are being provided are preferred or even necessary. To better understand the validity services that are being prescribed hundreds of thousands of times each day, it is important to better understand the general concept of variation and the science behind its analysis.

In 1988, John E. "Jack" Wennberg founded the Center for the Evaluative Sciences at Dartmouth College with the express purpose of better understanding the decisions that are made when determining whether a health-care service was to be provided.[83] Designed to support the overarching mission of Dartmouth College's Institute for Health Policy and Clinical Practices, its early mission was to improve health care through education, research, policy reform, leadership improvement, and communication with patients and the public.[84] As part of the institute's research and educational interests, the institute began publishing the *Dartmouth Atlas*, which explores the glaring variation in health-care service utilization driven largely by provider preferences reflecting geographic factors.[85] As a means of assessing service delivery efficiency and effectiveness at the level of a local community, a state, or a region of the country, the *Atlas* has been used by health-care researchers, policy makers, and local health systems to better assess the impact of changing practices.

80 G. F. Anderson, P. S. Hussey, B. K. Frogner, and H. R. Waters, "Health Spending in the United States and the Rest of the Industrialized World," *Health Affairs* 24, no. 4 (2005): 903–914.

81 J. Kane, "Health Costs: How the U.S. Compares with Other Countries," *PBS Newshour: The Rundown*, October 22, 2012, accessed May 15, 2017, http://www.pbs.org/newshour/rundown/health-costs-how-the-us-compares-with-other-countries/..

82 The Commonwealth Fund, "U.S. Health Care from a Global Perspective," October 8, 2015, accessed May 15, 2017, http://www.commonwealthfund.org/publications/issue-briefs/2015/oct/us-health-care-from-a-global-perspective.

83 "Dartmouth Medical Milestones," Dartmouth Geisel School of Medicine, accessed May 15, 2017, http://geiselmed.dartmouth.edu/about/milestones/.

84 The Dartmouth Institute for Health Policy & Clinical Practice, accessed March 15, 2017, http://tdi.dartmouth.edu/research.

85 *The Dartmouth Atlas*, accessed March 15, 2017, http://tdi.dartmouth.edu/research/evaluating/health-system-focus/the-dartmouth-atlas.

Multiple factors have been identified as having played a significant role in regional differences for medical spending, with many factors directly related to individual physician decision-making when prescribing health-care services.

The Dartmouth team further contributed to the science of variation in 2010, when they published an analysis of regional differences in diagnostic practices, citing diagnostic test ordering variation as one of the most important contributors to unwarranted health-care costs.[86] As the group evaluated the number and types of diagnoses given to patients as they moved from region to region, isolating for any meaningful difference in health status, the researchers noticed that diagnostic practices varied significantly between regional health-care delivery teams, and payments for services were directly influenced by the number and types of tests performed and the resulting diagnoses being generated, but seemed to be unrelated to individual patient characteristics. Since Medicare payments are based on the illness burden and functional status of patients, as additional diagnoses are rendered by a provider, billing and coding personnel then generate a claim for payment that reflects an increased patient illness burden, with higher reimbursement paid for the care provided for that individual. The results from this study demonstrated as much as a 52 percent difference between high-expense and low-expense providers for patients with nearly identical illness burdens.

With careful subanalysis, the research team also found that variation in administrative processes, such as diagnosis coding, produced significant variation in patient invoices submitted for Medicare payment. These types of analyses have helped shine a light on the widespread geographic variation in Medicare spending that was a key discussion point during the health-care policy debate in 1993 when the Clinton Health Plan was being launched, during the 2008 debate on the Affordable Care Act, and in March 2017 when a repeal-and-replace approach gave rise to the American Health Care Act proposed by House Majority Leader Paul Ryan. Many have suggested that if medical service delivery variability and coding-related risk adjustment bias

---

86 Y. Song et al., "Regional Variation in Diagnostic Practices," *New England Journal of Medicine* 363, no. 1 (2010): 45–62.

could be controlled, health-care costs could be made more manageable under any type of national health-care policy.

In an article appearing in 2010, Zhang and associates used Medicare data to assess the impact and origins of variation in Medicare drug spending.[87] After adjusting for local price-level differences and individual-level demographics such as age, race, and sex, the researchers analyzed variation in the medical and pharmaceutical spending for each of the 306 hospital referral areas as outlined in the methods used by the *Dartmouth Atlas*. Citing four specific reasons for local variation in pharmacy spending, the group demonstrated that even though drug spending does vary by geographic region, it appears to be unrelated to either medical-services spending or individual differences between patients. From this study, it appears that variation impacts not only the medical services being recommended by health-care providers but also the number and types of pharmaceutical agents being prescribed.

To better understand the reasons behind variation in prescribing medical services and pharmaceutical services, it is essential to understand the many factors leading to variation and to appreciate that variation can be "warranted" and can lead to improvements in care quality for an individual, while other types of variation are best described as "unwarranted," producing little positive benefit to a patient and even resulting in lower-quality patient care outcomes. Warranted variation typically is associated with patient-related factors such as the values-driven choices of a patient or the complexities of care related to comorbid conditions that may lead to a higher individual disease burden. Unwarranted variation in care is typically due to provider preferences that have little or no evidentiary support and produce systematic inefficiencies in care provision. The latter desire for delivering the correct number of services needed is typified by what many have called the "Goldilocks effect," where services delivered are not too many (lower levels of quality related to overuse errors), not too few (lower levels of quality related to underuse error), but are, rather, the precise number of services needed to produce a favorable clinical outcome. A CEO colleague of mine challenged his quality-improvement

---

87 Y. Zhang, K. Baicker, and J. P. Newhouse, "Geographic Variation in Medicare Drug Spending," *New England Journal of Medicine* 363, no. 5 (2010): 405–408.

teams to find care solutions that would "do the right thing the first time and every time" as a mental model aimed at promoting appropriate service delivery.

Provider-related variation in service delivery is a problem that has dogged health-care delivery systems for years. In a publication in 2014, Ballard explored the phenomenon of variation in service delivery that dates back at least to 1938 when Dr. J. Allison Glover found that the geographic variation in number of tonsillectomy procedures performed in England was directly tied to provider preference rather than to a patient's demonstrated need for services.[88] Some degree of service variation is always to be anticipated between regions since medical education, residency and fellowship training, and peer-to-peer learning do vary based on issues such as availability of new technology in one region compared to another. Other factors that can influence variation include imprecise medical literature that reduces the applicability of national approaches to systematic thinking, differences in knowledge diffusion rates between regions, and the presence of differing patient expectations that may be quite variable due to local culture.

Despite these caveats, most variation appears to be largely tied to individual provider behaviors, and the costs associated with these provider decisions may drive health-care spending differences.[89] While some have advocated for reimbursement reductions in regions where costs are statistically at odds with those of more moderate-cost regions, most policy makers understand that this may penalize patients with significant illness burdens who would be adversely affected by downregulating typical diagnostic testing patterns by providers in that area. A more prudent approach, many quality researchers believe, would be to disseminate provider education more broadly, coupled with a payment process for high-frequency conditions that would bundle the costs of

88 D. J. Ballard, B. Graca, et al., "Variation in Medical Practice and Implications for Quality," in *The Healthcare Quality Book: Vision, Strategy, and Tools*, 3rd ed., ed. Maulik S. Joshi, Elizabeth Ransom, David B. Nash, and Scott B. Ransom (Chicago, IL: Health Administration Press), 55–82.

89 L. L. Leape et al., "Does Inappropriate Use Explain Geographic Variations in the Use of Health Care Services? A Study of Three Procedures," *Journal of the American Medical Association* 263, no. 5 (1990): 669–672.

diagnostic testing, treatment, and follow-up services as a single payment to be divided among all providers engaged in service delivery.[90]

One campaign launched to reduce unwarranted variation in testing and treatment is the Choosing Wisely Campaign, sponsored by the American Board of Internal Medicine Foundation in conjunction with Consumer Reports.[91] Seeking to advance a national dialogue to reduce waste associated with unnecessary testing and ineffective treatments and procedures, the program calls on all medical and surgical specialties to identify commonly performed tests and procedures that those specialty societies feel to be most likely to suffer from overuse based on validated research. The campaign's supporters call for provider specialists to choose wisely when ordering tests and procedures, with the hope that only those services that are truly necessary and supported by evidence would be deployed to produce better clinical outcomes without harm. A listing by specialty society of tests that are most likely used in error has been provided, and many quality-improvement programs at hospitals and health systems use these lists as starting points for service utilization conversations with their medical staff.

An example of one such recommendation is related to the performance of expensive radiology testing for patients with uncomplicated low-back pain within the first six weeks of onset of pain. After excluding serious conditions such as nerve entrapment and infections in the spine, it was felt appropriate to begin symptomatic treatment for low-back pain without performing any diagnostic imaging studies, such as magnetic resonance imaging (MRI). Since low-back pain is the fifth-most common condition seen in office practices, and since MRI tests are very expensive, following the Choosing Wisely recommendations can produce very significant reductions in unwarranted variation and health-care spending.[92] At a former organization in which I worked, use

90 Centers for Medicare and Medicaid Services, "Bundled Payments for Care Improvement (BPCI) Initiative: General Information," accessed May 15, 2017, https://innovation.cms.gov/initiatives/bundled-payments/.

91 "Choosing Wisely: An Initiative of the ABIM Foundation," accessed May 15, 2017, http://www.choosingwisely.org/.

92 "Choosing Wisely: Back Pain Tests and Treatments," accessed May 15, 2017, http://www.choosingwisely.org/wp-content/uploads/2016/04/ChoosingWiselyBackPainAAMPR-ER.pdf.

of the campaign's recommendations on testing for back pain, coupled with education and data feedback loops for physicians that demonstrated their radiology testing utilization patterns versus those of their peers, helped change the evaluation process for low-back pain throughout the entire health system, yielding significant financial impact.

While unwarranted utilization can produce health-care costs that add layers of expense without adding commensurate improvements in quality, care processes can also be altered to generate higher-value care for consumers and health-care service payers. Several effective tactics have been used to generate more effective and efficient care systems, and while many focus on provider behavior, it is important to note that in this era of consumerism, many improvement efforts are also aimed at addressing individual patient preferences and behaviors. The first improvement tactic is simply to gather all interested parties together to agree on the goals for the changes to be implemented. These goals illustrate the changes in practice needed to produce clinical enhancements, including metrics of total cost of care and documentation of the impact on the patient experience. Developing such a comprehensive set of measures brings the community of care providers and care consumers into a more highly aligned relationship, allowing results to be demonstrated for all participants in the care experience, and it promotes joint contributions toward ongoing modifications should these measures of success not trend in a favorable direction. Available technology such as electronic health records with decision support tools can help clinicians and their patients stick to an evidence-based approach to testing and treatment of common health conditions. Care processes should be constructed using input from all team participants, and small tests of change need to be piloted before implementing permanent changes in the care experience. Data and feedback loops need to be made available to both providers and consumers of care so that changes can be made that reflect the joint decision-making preferences of both providers and consumers. Finally, since this improvement step implies participation in a very human process, efforts should be made to attend to high-reliability science with a focus on human resiliency.[93]

93 T. Granzyk, "Resilience in Healthcare. The Doctor Weighs In," June 29, 2013, accessed May 15, 2017, https://thedoctorweighsin.com/resilience-in-healthcare/.

This focus is quite different from other industries, such as manufacturing, where an approach to standardizing a process views variation as mostly predictable and unwarranted, since the substrate used in production is typically inorganic, involving the interaction between materials and machines. In health care, where human variation can occur simply due to the unique ways in which humans differ from one another, resilient systems with a focus on unpredictable events that may arise need to be implemented to better recover from defects explicitly related to the human condition. Systematic process improvements that pay special attention to key care process steps that alter the care outcome and are based solely on the human interface are one way to enhance system effectiveness. An example of this type of attention to the human substrate can be seen when care managers and patient navigators collaborate closely to monitor critical decision points in a treatment plan, focusing on early recognition of variation in individual care responses that may arise in some patients.

Health systems are becoming more deliberate in their efforts aimed at reducing unwarranted variation that leads to overuse of services. Both rewards and penalties have recently created significant financial focus for health systems, including incentives to report quality metrics and the implementation of penalties for excessive utilization and untoward clinical outcomes such as hospital-acquired conditions (HACs) and readmission to the hospital following treatment. These changes in payment practices are directed at creating rewards for higher-value care practices where health-care providers are beginning to assume financial risk for managing patients when they use strategies that promote greater care process efficiency and effectiveness. Hospitals are now even advertising price and service guarantees as they look to minimize process waste and deliver health outcomes that are visibly different from their competitors.

One such model, established by Geisinger Health System based in rural Danbury, Pennsylvania, incorporates evidence-based health practices that have been demonstrated through research to be most effective.[94] By determining

---

94 D. McCarthy, K. Mueller, and Wrenn, Issues Research Inc., "Geisinger Health System: Achieving the Potential of System Integration through Innovation, Leadership, Measurement,

the key medical practices most associated with a favorable outcome for car-diovascular surgery, Geisinger standardized care and measured process varia-tion to perfect the health-care experience of open heart surgery. Labeling the approach ProvenCare, the health system rapidly expanded from improve-ments in heart surgery to other service lines that also would benefit from such predictable approaches. Treating ProvenCare as a service guarantee, Geisinger promoted these practices in contracts with health insurers, promising that if costs exceeded what was expected from the guaranteed approaches, the health system would bear any incremental costs associated with additional services needed to correct defects. The program has been highly successful financially, and it has also enhanced patient confidence that they are receiving the highest-quality care. A variety of metrics have been used to demonstrate success, includ-ing reduced length of hospital stay, reduced readmission rates, reduced rates of hospital-based infections, and in-hospital mortality rates driven to zero for the conditions under study. In short, the ProvenCare approach benefits health-care consumers, providers, and payers through simple and extremely focused care practices that reinforce the application of evidence-based approaches to the daily care of each of the health system's patients.

Practices such as those deployed at Geisinger are taking hold throughout the country, but health systems that are attempting to reduce clinical varia-tion have required novel systems to support these efforts. Incorporated into hospital quality and clinical effectiveness departments, these support services are typically described as "care management services" or "care coordination services." While opportunities to improve system effectiveness and efficiency may vary from region to region, there are some health conditions that dem-onstrate transcendent opportunities for improvement in service coordination. These conditions include the treatment of chronic health-care conditions such as heart failure and diabetes, high-risk surgical procedures, advanced care planning, and care for patients who are transitioning between various levels

and Incentives," The Commonwealth Fund: Case Study, June 2009, accessed May 15, 2017, http://www.commonwealthfund.org/~/media/Files/Publications/Case%20Study/2009/Jun/McCarthy_Geisinger_case_study_624_update.pdf..

of service such as from the hospital to skilled nursing home environments. Falling under the flag of Care Management Services are five key elements that all must work together for more effective and efficient care patterns to be demonstrated for a growing number of high-complexity patients with unique care needs.

The first component of the new Care Management model, a holdover from early days of health insurance financial controls, is called Utilization Management Services. Patients with extended hospital stays that exceed what had been predicted are candidates for utilization management oversight. Specially trained hospital staff use a variety of length-of-stay predictive tools to help manage the financial consequences of each patient being admitted. These tools match the number of days typically expected to be needed to treat common health conditions against the expected reimbursement for those conditions, and as patients begin to exceed their "expected length of stay," utilization personnel work closely with inpatient treatment teams to assess whether a patient might be able to be discharged to a lower-cost service level such as a nursing home or even home with assistance. Evaluation of patients by utilization management staff is based on a patient's medical necessity for services, and discussions about discharge are held with treatment teams, patient families, and hospital finance teams. These discussions can often be quite strained, as patient placement at the most appropriate level of service is interpreted by some patients and families as being solely financially motivated. Utilization specialists typically have clinical or social-work backgrounds and have adapted unique communication skills that are needed to implement a discharge plan with sensitivity to the patient's needs and the patient family's preferences.

The second component of Care Management is Case Management, which assists in developing an integrated and collaborative treatment plan for a small subset of patients who are felt to be at highest risk of having a poor health outcome, largely due to the number and intensity of clinical conditions present in these high-complexity patients. Intensive care plans that call for individually tailored approaches to care and longitudinal follow-up make the job of the case manager quite difficult, as unique solutions to individual patient problems can be profound in their impact. An example of how case managers come to the assistance of high-risk patients is in managing patients with end-stage kidney disease due to diabetes, where special efforts need to be focused on relatively simple care needs such as meal preparation, self-administration of insulin in individuals who may have significant visual impairment, transportation from home to a dialysis facility three or four times per week, making arrangements for screening for a kidney transplant evaluation, and myriad other services and appointments that need to be individually coordinated and monitored for effectiveness.

A third component of Care Management is Disease Management Services, where a narrow focus is given to care plans for patients suffering from specific diseases where certain interventions will be needed on an ongoing basis. Coordination of care with a disease management specialist has been demonstrated to produce favorable outcomes such as reduction in hospital admissions and visits to the emergency department or urgent-care clinics to manage a sudden clinical decompensation related to a specific disease. Examples of conditions that have been favorably managed using disease management tactics include asthma, early stages of diabetes, and high blood pressure where evidence-based approaches have been shown to be very effective in reducing the frequency with which clinical episodes of disease decompensation occur. Not only do these negative outcomes affect cost of care, but they also signal systematic failure of treatment planning or care execution and lead to erosion of patient confidence in a system to which they have entrusted their care.

The fourth component of Care Management is labeled Clinical Standardization, which involves assistance from a specialized set of clinicians who design specific evidence-based approaches to be deployed by disease managers and utilization managers. These administrative supports are typically applied in the ambulatory care environment, and they involve experts who review the medical literature and endorse and introduce care pathways that reflect the most up-to-date care plans that are relevant to ambulatory sites of service. Targeted approaches to diagnosis and treatment of common conditions are the strength of clinical standardization experts, and the tools typically employed follow recommendations from best practices that include the rollout of educational programs for provider teams, data displays that demonstrate variation in practice of providers, and the use of electronic health record tools such as clinical decision support that hardwires the consistent use of best practices in daily care.

Finally, Care Management teams include Patient Engagement specialists, whose job is to consistently build communication bridges between patients and families and the care teams. Using outreach and educational methods, engagement specialists ensure that patients and their families continue to remain invested in the prescribed care plan while also promoting self-care for many aspects of their treatment plan. One of the greatest contributions made by engagement specialists is the follow-through on treatment plans and the adherence to medication strategies. By engaging patients and their families in discussions about the use of medications, adherence to life-sustaining medications can be enhanced, leading to longer-term clinical stabilization and a reduced need for higher-cost services should medication strategies fail. Due to emerging high-complexity medical strategies, patients may have difficulty understanding the reasons for initiation of a new medication, misunderstand the benefits and side effects of a medication, and have questions regarding the purchase of these medications in a stressful financial climate where chronic disease can cause patients to choose whether to consistently take a medication or to meet other financial obligations such as paying rent or buying food.

The complexity of providing care to and for a patient with multiple diseases is challenging, and the number of support staff surrounding such an individual can create confusion for patients and their families, placing a unique strain on the provider-patient relationship. A frequent complaint from a person interacting with so many partners on a treatment team is that it is unclear exactly who is fulfilling the role of the initial point of contact, the so-called responsible agent for directing care. Frequent handoffs of the responsibility for care decisions are typically experienced, leaving patients wondering about the most appropriate person to turn to if they are having difficulty understanding or adhering to a component of their individualized care plans. Further complicating the relationships with the care provider team is understanding the predicament faced by health-care consumers as they interface with those who are responsible for administering payment for health-care services, the health insurance companies. With a vested interest in the way in which funds are to be efficiently disbursed to provide care for their beneficiaries, health insurance payers play a specialized role of providing fiduciary oversight for patient care that is sometimes interpreted by providers and consumers as being at odds with meeting the goals of a treatment plan aimed at how best to fulfill the care needs of a patient.

As health systems have evolved to manage the greater number of payment relationships arising from more complex private and governmental payment plans, a cottage industry has also sprung up to support providers and consumers of care. When government payers shifted to an inpatient prospective payment system (IPPS) that was based on the sum total of the illness burden of a patient receiving services in a hospital setting, accuracy of information being provided by the hospital to the government became paramount.[95] To guarantee prompt payment for invoices submitted for payment, health systems have developed sophisticated billing and coding processes that capture data from the medical record and translate those data into billing codes. The greater the number of codes and the greater intensity of services that are supported by these diagnostic codes, the greater the reimbursement that will be received under fixed payment methodologies. Diagnosis codes can be modified when patients have multiple diagnoses or when they suffer from complications related to their original condition, and these billing codes are further subclassified as routine or majorly complicating. When clinical data support the presence of a coexisting medical condition, hospital-employed coders capture this information to support the fact that a patient had much higher-complexity care needs that required additional care resources during hospitalization, driving the billing codes toward greater reimbursement.

An example of such coding is the presence of a patient with heart failure admitted to the hospital for management of pneumonia. Treatment of relatively uncomplicated patients with pneumonia can be assumed to require

95 Centers for Medicare and Medicaid Services, "Acute Inpatient PPS," accessed May 16, 2017, https://www.cms.gov/Medicare/Medicare-Fee-for-Service-Payment/AcuteInpatientPPS/index.html.

a standardized set of resources such as antibiotics, oxygen, and monitoring by a nursing team, with periodic X-rays and laboratory testing to document clinical progress. If a patient is admitted to the hospital for treatment of pneumonia but also suffers from long-standing heart failure, additional resources would be needed, such as specialized heart monitoring and medications to treat heart failure in addition to the antibiotics and oxygen needed for pneumonia therapy. This greater set of resources raises the expense incurred by the hospital to treat the patient, and hospital coders accurately capture this coexistent heart failure condition to generate a billing invoice reflecting the new level of service intensity needed to treat pneumonia. Counterbalancing this additional coding is a relatively new set of rules that are tied to penalties in reimbursement should the hospital stay produce a complication directly tied to the treatment of the patient. One such example of this is the negative impact to reimbursement seen when a complication is encountered following a procedure or if a patient develops inpatient bedsores where routine nutrition, physical therapy, and bed positioning of the patient may have prevented such a complication. These complications, called "hospital acquired conditions" (HACs), are patient safety events that are viewed as avoidable and therefore not reimbursed by payers. These events also appear in public reports on hospital quality and safety and have a negative impact on any reimbursement bonuses paid by federal payers.

One further resource employed by hospitals to assist clinical teams in their efforts to safely and effectively deliver care to patients is the information found in the electronic medical record that helps uncover and implement best clinical practices. While this will be more thoroughly explored in a subsequent chapter, it should also be captured in discussions about the hospital methods used to transform and improve care practices. The electronic health record is a library of all patient-level information including diagnostic data such as the tests ordered, therapeutic interventions made, and prognostic outlook, expressed by each member of the treatment team. Historically, these data have been difficult to capture in a succinct and useful fashion, and many patients have suffered due to a lack of a consistent approach to data capture that promotes an integrated assessment of a patient's care plan. With the ascent of electronic health records, key advantages seen from more highly integrated care have emerged, and a more thorough accounting of a patient's clinical challenges has helped the care team become more efficient and effective in their daily efforts to deliver on a promise of better health-care practices that translate into a better quality of life for a patient.

To what end has the proliferation of hospital teams promoted stronger relationships between care teams, patients, and families? On the positive side, capturing the person's values-driven care preferences has helped reduce the number of undesired services provided on behalf of persons who may not have previously expressed their wishes. This is especially important when patients and families have already voiced a preference for a specific medical intervention. Some of the more important examples of these preadmission decisions include whether the treatment team should use electrical shock or medications to attempt to restart a person's heart if it were to stop suddenly or if a person wishes to have a breathing tube inserted when there is little chance for meaningful recovery from an unrelenting disease such as terminal cancer or end-stage kidney disease. Having this information available to a treatment team allows them to fulfill the exact preferences of a patient, customizing the care plan.

Well-designed care management teams can help patients and their loved ones ensure that services appropriate to the patient's desires are used both in the hospital and following hospital discharge, when high-complexity conditions may make a patient's transition to a different level of service quite tenuous. The most important conversations with patients and their families often center on the availability of outpatient support services that can fulfill a treatment plan that was initiated in the hospital setting. Services such as home care, nutrition support in the form of meals on wheels, and physical therapy can be arranged by the care coordinator to help provide the most appropriate services in the correct setting. By paying attention to an individual's personal preferences, a care experience can be created that is highly customized to the patient. These hospital support services have been typically well received by patients and families and have also been well received by all members of the care team so that a care plan is deployed that is more likely to meet the personal goals of the health-care consumer.

On the flip side, care management services are seen as intrusive by some care providers and care consumers. In these settings, care teams can complain that "someone who does not understand what needs to be done for the patient is watching over my shoulder," and some patients have expressed a concern that they are being "driven out of the hospital before they are ready for discharge." These comments reflect their views about the relatively new addition of business services and insurance into the sacred space of a provider-consumer relationship. What had been previously a very personal and individual bond is now part of a larger group conversation where a person's customized treatment plan becomes modified by newly added care team members. Further complicating this relationship is the perception that these new team members are primarily focused on how best to maximize the financial value of the care transaction.

Key Points to Master From Chapter 6

- Health care costs are driven by the number of services utilized multiplied by the cost of each individual service. Both need to be addressed in health care finance reform.
- The United States spends a greater percent of its GDP compared to other industrialized nations; quality and safety results do not match these investments.
- Variations in care practices may be either "warranted" when they lead to improvements in care quality for an individual while other types of variation are described as "unwarranted" when they produce little positive benefit to a patient or when they result in lower quality patient care outcomes. Warranted variation typically is associated with patient-related factors such as the values-driven choices made by patients or significant complexities of care related to co-morbid conditions. Unwarranted variations in care are due to provider preferences that have little or no evidentiary support or to systematic inefficiencies in care provision.
- The Choosing Wisely Campaign® asks provider specialties to identify and eliminate tests and treatments that are not evidence-based.
- Health systems are responding to public reporting of quality and safety measures, coupled with financial incentives, to reduce unwarranted variation. ProvenCare® is an example of how providers are offering price guarantees for their adherence to evidence-based guidelines for care.
- Components of care management services that help to secure the needed services delivered by the most appropriate clinician at the correct time in a care experience include:
  - Utilization Management – identifies expected length of stay
  - Case Management – develops an integrated treatment plan
  - Disease Management – applies specific disease treatment protocols

- o Clinical Standardization – develops evidence-based pathways of care
- o Patient Engagement Specialists – promotes application of a person's values to the care being experienced.

Seven

THE IMPACT OF QUALITY AND SAFETY SYSTEMS

W hen the Institute of Medicine (IOM) announced in late 1999 that as many as ninety-eight thousand people die each year as a result of the faulty care practices found in the American health-care delivery system, the report sent shock waves throughout the country.[96] Providers of care pushed back, stating that the data had been extrapolated using unscientific methods, while health-care consumers wanted an explanation for how the "best health care in the world" could produce such terrifying consequences. In patient surveys carried out that year in my health-care organization, it came as no surprise that patients identified personal safety as the most important item of concern when they were admitted to the hospital. To put perspective on the numbers that were being bandied about, deaths related to medical error exceeded the raw death figures from motor-vehicle accidents, breast cancer, and HIV/AIDS combined,[97] and the reputational cost to American hospitals from a perception of daily delivery of unsafe health care was unprecedented. With both providers and consumers in shock, the safety movement was launched in United States

---

96 Linda T. Kohn, Janet M. Corrigan, and Molla S. Donaldson, eds., *To Err Is Human. Building a Safer Health System* (Washington, DC: National Academy Press, 1999).

97 Centers for Disease Control and Prevention (National Center for Health Statistics), "Births and Deaths: Preliminary Data for 1998," *National Vital Statistics Reports* 47, no. 25 (1999): 6.

health care, while medical administrators attempted to document improvements that had been put in place to enhance the quality of services provided that would make care experiences predictably safer and of higher value.

Not only did the IOM publication identify the clinical and reputational impact resulting from less safe care, it also pointed out the financial toll that was being taken from these same faulty processes. Clearly identified in a discussion regarding the true costs of low-quality care were the incremental costs resulting from ineffective care plans, costs associated with additional tests and treatments needed to restore health to patients who had been injured by the delivery system, and malpractice expenses resulting from poor health outcomes that arose when patients and providers were exposed to low-quality care processes. Perhaps the biggest shock to everyone reading the report was the historic silence that had enveloped health-care safety for years. Both providers and consumers of care had long assumed that high levels of quality and safety could be relegated to simple afterthoughts, since these foundational elements were already built into the care experience.

Not only had safety concerns been finally drawn into the open, but the discussion also turned to the many ways that health care had been overstating its basic levels of quality. The institute's follow-up publication on American health-care quality in 2001 was equally scathing regarding safety practices.[98] From its initial sentence, the report's authors from the Committee on the Quality of Health Care in America stated explicitly that "the American health care delivery system is in need of fundamental change." The report uncovered an unpleasant fact: that Americans were not receiving care that would meet their needs based on the best scientific knowledge available, and there existed a chasm between the health care that we have and the care we should have. Similar to its initial report on health-care safety, the Institute of Medicine identified defects in care delivery system processes, outlining specific tactics that needed to begin immediately to satisfy the promise made to all Americans that this country's health-care systems should deliver outcomes that exceeded those found in the rest of the industrialized world. Acknowledging that science

---

98 William C. Richardson, chair, *Crossing the Quality Chasm: A New Health System for the 21ˢᵗ Century* (Washington, DC: National Academy Press, 2001).

and technology had advanced at a rapid pace, the committee found that high-quality care was being delivered inconsistently and that there was great variability in health system performance that could not be explained solely due to characteristics of health-care consumers found in a particular region. Drawing an analogy that health care in the last quarter of the twentieth century was best seen as part of an "era of Brownian motion," the report likened health-care quality improvement to the random motion of particles where some improvements were being seen, but there was no predictable pattern that could be documented as having been responsible for systematic and logical change.[99]

The questions arising from the Institute of Medicine observations were challenging and disturbing, but the reports provided significant impetus for hospitals across the country to become more deeply engaged in implementing tactics that could demonstrate the resolve needed to design safety and quality into daily patient care processes. Before discussing the impact of quality and safety defects on the provider-consumer compact, it is important to understand a few of the reasons for the inertia that had been uncovered in the quality and safety reports, beginning with a discussion regarding the psychology of health-care providers and their inability to engage in systematic improvement efforts.

When Everett M. Rogers first published his treatise on how innovations diffuse through groups,[100] he cited studies from Ryan and Gross that outlined the barriers to change experienced in the early efforts to promote the use of hybrid seed corn in Iowa.[101] Midwestern farmers had been exposed to a more drought-resistant and hearty new seed corn, but the slow uptake of its use concerned many agricultural experts who felt that the hybrid seed's higher cost might be the sole determinant of poor adoption practices. Analyzing the data from surveys conducted by Ryan and Gross, Rogers was able to identify basic human factors that were responsible for the uneven adoption of a superior

---

99 Albert Einstein, *Investigations on the Theory of the Brownian Movement* (Dover Publications, 1956).

100 E. M. Rogers, *Diffusion of Innovations*, 5th ed. (New York: Free Press, 2003, originally published 1962).

101 B. Ryan and N. C. Gross, "The Diffusion of Hybrid Seed Corn in Two Iowa Communities," *Rural Sociology* 8 (1943): 15–24.

technology, and the model he proposed became associated with what is called Rogers's change model for human behavior. His observations identified some farmers who immediately implemented the improved corn-growing methods using the new seed corn hybrids, while others waited to monitor the initial results from the so-called early adopters. Still others lagged behind for years until they nearly suffered economic collapse from having not adopted new farming methods earlier.

Human factors such as risk tolerance, a desire for factual input, the inability to adopt changes based on preliminary successes, and a fear of making errors in judgment are responsible for the uneven adoption patterns in farming practices seen by Rogers, and they are also true of providers in American health-care delivery systems. There appears to be relatively slow and uneven adoption of the process changes needed to produce improvements in health-care quality and safety practices that can generate more favorable and predictable outcomes. When Coleman and colleagues published results of a study on physician adoption of a newly released antibiotic in 1966, the importance of strong interpersonal networking was demonstrated from the observation that more tightly networked physicians tended to use the new medication faster than those physicians who were less engaged with their medical colleagues.[102] Use of the antibiotic called "gammanym" was studied over a period of seventeen months, and rates of adoption by internists, general practitioners, and pediatricians were studied. The investigators found that 15 percent of physicians had used the drug by the end of two months and 50 percent had used the new medication by the end of six months, but there were still 25 percent of physicians who had not used the new drug even after ten months following its release for widespread use by all physicians. Following the same general S-shaped curve that had been described in Rogers's earlier work, it appeared that physicians' adoption of new techniques and methods represented the same social networking principles as Iowa farmers' adoption of hybrid seed corn. Some physicians were labeled early adopters of innovative care practices and were responsible for pulling their colleagues along to change

---

102 J. S. Coleman, E. Katz, and H. Menzel, *Medical Innovation: A Diffusion Study* (The Bobbs-Merrill Company, 1966), 25–37.

practice patterns, while other providers were noted to adopt new methods at much slower rates. A small but significant group, representing approximately 15 percent of practitioners, could be labeled as "laggards" due to their delayed adoption of innovative technologies and treatments.

Rogers outlined a variety of reasons for the decision-making speed of people who take a more cautious approach to adopting new technologies. Acknowledging that there existed a strong quality-control concern that could be logically used to prevent harm from early adoption of faulty science, Rogers suggested that consensus development conferences by groups such as the Food and Drug Administration (FDA) could be assembled to give late adopters comfort that experts had evaluated the new method for efficacy and safety, and to identify potentially unintended consequences resulting from early adoption. A counterbalancing force suggests that delays in getting new medications to market may prevent new cures from becoming incorporated into mainstream medical care, and that laggards are directly responsible for taking too cautious an approach to these innovative strategies.[103]

Rogers has described five key stages for adoption of innovation starting with the stage of new *knowledge acquisition*, when a person is first exposed to a new process or product and yet is not inspired enough to learn more about a new idea to adopt its use. This is followed by a *persuasion* phase, in which the individual becomes interested in finding out more, followed by the most variable phase of *decision*, where the individual weighs the benefits and risks to decide whether to adopt or reject the new proposal. The final two phases include *implementation*, where an individual variably utilizes the new method, technique, or product to assess its preliminary impact, and the final phase of *confirmation*, where the individual uses interpersonal conversations with others to affirm and finalize the wisdom of adopting the new method. Frustrating to many is the delay in adopting new techniques that may be uniquely positioned to save lives and present new safety improvement opportunities for health-care practices. Writing in the *New Yorker*, Dr. Atul Gawande, a prolific author and observer of physician behavior change, noted that health care is

---

103 S. Kazman, "Drug Approvals and Deadly Delays," *Journal of Americans Physicians and Surgeons* 15, no. 4 (2010): 101–103.

still trying to find a way to introduce twentieth-century methods into the twenty-first century of medical practices.[104]

Many health-care organizations have created focused interventions designed to enhance the rates of adoption of new methods by their medical practitioners. One such organization, Wesley Medical Center in Wichita, Kansas, has implemented team communication tools labeled TeamSTEPPS[105] (Team Strategies & Tools to Enhance Performance & Patient Safety) to educate its physicians by following a strategy arising from Kotter's Eight Step Process for Leading Change[106] to promote better communication regarding the improvement tools that they wish to put in place. As a more formal communications approach was used, improvement in safety metrics could be documented in the health system's public reports, supporting the claim that higher degrees of safety and quality could be obtained from making their care processes more intentional while reinforcing the new communications methods during each encounter.

Designing and deploying health-care processes that embrace greater degrees of quality and safety is certainly not an easy task for most hospitals and health systems. When high-value health care was initially described by the Institute of Medicine, the committee proposed six main determinants (the Six Aims) that are used as care principles seen in high-performing systems. These included care practices that reinforced safer care, provided more timely access to services, adopted care processes that were both effective and efficient, and delivered care that was patient-centered and equitable for all.[107] Since it was determined that many paths could lead to the same result, the committee did not prescribe a specific quality-improvement method to be used by everyone. The most important IOM findings included a call to overcome inertia, and

---

104 A. Gawande, "Slow Ideas," *The New Yorker*, July 29, 2013.

105 TeamSTEPPS, Agency for Healthcare Research and Quality, accessed March 17, 2017, https://www.ahrq.gov/teamstepps/webinars/index.html.

106 Kotter International, accessed March 17, 2017, https://www.kotterinternational.com/8-steps-process-for-leading-change/.

107 Committee on Quality of Health Care in America, Institute of Medicine, *Crossing the Quality Chasm: A New Health System for the 21ˢᵗ Century* (Washington, DC: National Academy Press, 2001).

the only way to achieve the final care process goal was to begin improvement efforts immediately and at the earliest point in every care process. Borrowing from James Collins's work on organizational change,[108] the committee provided a call to action for US health-care delivery systems by suggesting that systems not let perfection stand in the way of taking steps to build better health-care delivery processes.

There are many reasons why health systems have difficulty in changing their basic constructs for quality and safety, and many of these are unrelated to the individual human behavioral reasons to resist change. As practices have become deeply entrenched from years of repetition, they begin to develop a self-reinforcing sense of validity and status. For great health systems to evolve, they need to abandon many of these perceived notions and begin to explore whether care services are being delivered in a fashion that meets the expectations set by the Institute of Medicine through the Six Aims. Health systems have approached the growing complexity of care by relying on individual expertise of their clinicians to define the practice patterns for those institutions, sometimes at the expense of embracing newer methods that are evidence-based and validated by multiple other organizations. Opportunities to identify systematic solutions are also frequently missed when organizations support highly customized approaches that do not incorporate organization-wide learning. In some cases, evidence-based practices and national benchmarks are lacking, leading to individual practitioners developing permissive clinical autonomy where the search for standardized approaches to care is abandoned. Finally, many organizations lack formal structures to incorporate reliability science into their efforts. As random practices become the standard for some organizations, four major defects in learning theory are proffered to obviate an ongoing need to develop more disciplined approaches to implementing evidence-based practices.[109]

---

108 J. C. Collins, *Good to Great: Why Some Companies Make the Leap...and Others Don't* (New York: HarperCollins, 2001).

109 R. Perla, "Health Care Reform and the Trap of the 'Iron Law,'" *Health Affairs Blog*, http://healthaffairs.org/blog.

The first of these defective practices is called the search for "cargo cult improvements." When organizations try to oversimplify solutions to complex conundrums, they are often guilty of attempting to implement fixed protocols that have not fully incorporated evidence-based change principles that are needed to be successful. During a 1974 commencement address to the graduates of the California Institute of Technology, physicist Richard Feynman introduced the term "cargo cult" to describe the ways in which prescientific cultures interpret technologically sophisticated visitors as being supernatural figures who bring "cargo" to enhance the economic conditions of a tribe. Seen in the South Pacific during World War II when American military installations delivered food, clothing, and other goods to tribal islands on which forward airbases were constructed, the islands still celebrate the rituals they believe were responsible for having those fruitful visits initiated in the 1940s. To return to the days when materials were given freely to the tribespeople by American airmen, islanders today continue construction and maintenance of airstrips, march in formation using bamboo sticks as rifles while simulating military formations, and use wood and bamboo to create headphones similar to those seen during the American occupation, all with the express purpose of reproducing the exact events that led up to the arrival of their supernatural visitors. Feynman cautioned against oversimplified solutions that could be deployed when one is fooled by abandoning deeper searches for reproducible success. Cargo cult solutions are often not long lasting or particularly accurate, since they do not expose the true barriers that need to be changed to create sustainable system quality. One specific example of the use of this defect in improvement thinking is in the use of checklists before surgical procedures. If the checklist is a simplified effort that has been put in place without understanding the underlying cultural aspects of team communication, then sustainable improvements are often lacking, and the potential for patient harm remains inherent in the system.

Another defect in quality thinking is that of "creating Fordlandia," named after the community created in Brazil by Henry Ford when he was attempting to enhance his automobile manufacturing empire.[110] By building an

---

110 J. Zasky, "Fordlandia: The Rise and Fall of Henry Ford's Forgotten Jungle City," *Failure Magazine*, June 21, 2009, accessed May 24, 2017, http://failuremag.com/article/fordlandia.

automobile assembly plant deep in the Amazon rain forest, Ford postulated that the new facility would be closer to a supply of rubber trees needed to produce tires for his cars. Without understanding the local context of the environment and its population, Ford identically reproduced an American city in the rain forest, complete with a requirement to use the same clothing, housing, and religious affiliations that were found in the United States. When cultural revolt ensued and rubber trees were destroyed due to insect infestations, the manufacturing plant was closed and labeled a massive failure. In health care, "one size fits all" approaches are frequently unsuccessful, since intricate details in cultural assimilation are not fully appreciated. An example of this is the difference between American and Australian health system results from implementation of rapid response teams (RRTs), designed to bring specialized treatment nurses to a patient's bedside in response to early signs of a patient's clinical deterioration.[111] In studies performed in the United States, RRTs were found to produce significant improvement in acute care outcomes, but when those same processes were studied abroad, no change in cardiac arrest, transfer to intensive care unit, or inpatient mortality was seen when compared to times before RRT adoption. As researchers began looking at the two comparison groups, it became obvious that the two clinical settings were quite different culturally, and simplified conclusions could not be drawn concerning the effectiveness of this new care process.

Diminishing returns can also be seen in quality efforts related to defects in the approach to implementation of new care processes.[112] When specific programs are rolled out that lack a set of principles and tactics needed to specifically and effectively implement a new process, sustainable adoption of these programs will be incomplete. Clarity of the methods used to implement key interventions in new process adoption can be more important than the process tactics themselves, similar to having a shiny new piece of technology

111 *K.* Hillman et al., "Introduction of the Medical Emergency Team (MET) System: A Cluster-Randomised Controlled Trial," *Lancet* 365, no. 9477: 2091–7.

112 L. J. Damschroder, "Fostering Implementation of Health Services Research Findings into Practice: A Consolidated Framework for Advancing Implementation Science," *Implementation Science* 4 (2009): 50, accessed March 17, 2017.

at one's disposal but lacking the handbook that describes the best uses of that technology. When scientific research documents the beneficial results from an intervention, it becomes essential for other organizations attempting similar improvements to be aware of the precise tools needed to manage the implementation efforts. Culture differences, use of alternative colloquial definitions or terminology, and availability of unique resources for deployment of such interventions are some of the most common implementation effort errors encountered.

The final error seen as organizations attempt to create an environment where changes can be introduced is in the human behavior of dogmatism, where rigid and fixed protocols are narrowly researched in a clinical context and do not translate perfectly well in a scalable and more generalized set of care environments. With even minor modifications that are not scrutinized as they are directly applied, generalized improvement is sometimes impossible to sustain since, like the Fordlandia errors, the context for implementation is of crucial importance. Overreliance on dogmatic solutions that do not reflect the culture of the implementing organization may create angst in early adopters who may slow or stop improvement efforts if process failures are seen that had not been anticipated. Without sensitivity to an organization's adoption culture, well-intentioned and evidence-based processes may be abandoned before any real opportunity to improve is ever realized.

With the many barriers to change and the vast number of ways in which implementation science defects may produce irregular improvement, how should an organization take initial steps to promote higher degrees of quality and patient safety that will benefit both providers and consumers of care? In addressing the new paradigm where health-care consumers are demanding to be included in the design of health-care improvement solutions, a blueprint is now generally available for how organizations can assemble more effective structures to implement change. Borrowing from other high-risk industries such as aviation, aerospace, and chemical engineering, health care is beginning to use the lessons learned from those sectors. Using improvement science design principles, health-care systems are producing more comprehensive solutions that reflect the values of all interested parties to focus on how they should create processes that meet the Six Aims of the Institute of Medicine, and by doing so, those systems help repair and reinforce the provider-consumer compact.

When Avedis Donabedian, one of the most prolific authors and a dedicated champion for the quality movement, proposed a framework in 1966 for evaluating the effectiveness of health-care improvement practices, he called for careful attention to "structure," "process," and "outcomes" as the essential components of the three-legged stool of improvement science.[113] To better understand the construct for how quality-improvement efforts are organized in health-care organizations, it is important to understand how the Donabedian model has been used to describe their construction (structure), how tools are used to enhance quality and safety results (process), and how results are measured and reported (outcomes).

Structure. As health-care systems begin to approach the creation of an effective structure for quality-improvement processes to be deployed, one essential element rises above all others. The most critical component of any improvement setting is finding a passionate leader for the new movement. This change agent begins to evaluate the organization honestly and systematically, reviewing the current state while looking outside the organization for exemplars that can assist in formulating an approach to change. This person is typically a clinician who is aware of the opportunities for improvement within the system and a person who feels passionately that the system can be improved. From a recent publication by Joshi, the clinician-leader has five key competencies that are essential to helping lead a fledgling quality and safety program.[114] Not only does the leader need to be an effective communicator of the vision of what health-care processes will look like following implementation of a quality structure, he or she must be capable of using data, have an interest in receiving inputs from both health-care providers and consumers, have some experience with building interdisciplinary teams, and understand

---

113 A. Donabedian, "The Quality of Care: How Can It Be Assessed?," *Journal of the American Medical Association* 260 (1988): 1743–1748, accessed March 17, 2017, https://jama.1988.03410120089033.

114 Joshi et al., *Leading Health Care Transformation.*

that the end product from these efforts should result in enhancements to the value of the health-care outcomes being delivered.

Typically, health system quality and safety programs have four essential and overarching components: quality control, quality improvement, quality personnel development, and quality innovation. This "four corners" approach generates an improvement model that can be easily visualized by health system governing boards, which are ultimately responsible for resourcing such programs while overseeing their sustainability. Quality control is typically the entry level to a quality and safety program and supports the monitoring results from existing practices, helping identify care processes that are most in need of improvement, while also documenting the outcomes of care processes that have longer track records of success. Seen predominantly as monitoring and auditing to standards, quality-control programs are fostered by organizations such as the Joint Commission, which issues standards for accreditation of health-care organizations, giving those organizations a blue-ribbon status for having met the minimum threshold of standards regarding their structures for care.[115] Quality-control efforts are largely aimed at meeting compliance measures and ensuring that the health-care organization has deployed the quality structures to audit care processes and to report variations in care when compared against a set of quality standards. Organizations that initiate quality-control programs have structures that are highly tactical in nature, are overseen by a few strong leaders, and have a focus on data collection that drives productivity standards.

As organizational efforts mature, alignment of care processes across multiple sites of service is noted, along with structures that promote physician leadership by employing one of their own to help lead the health system's quality programming.[116] Typically, when organizations predominantly focus on meeting accreditation standards, they may have error rates that range between one defect per one hundred care experiences to one defect per one thousand care experiences. Health-care organizations mature further when their structural

---

115 The Joint Commission webpage, accessed March 21, 2017, https://www.jointcommission.org/.

116 S. Dobbs and J. Reddy, *The 4 Phases of Quality Maturity* (Healthcare Financial Management Association, August 2011), 1–8.

approach shifts to supporting quality-improvement efforts instead of simply monitoring and auditing care processes. When moving into this phase of organizational maturity, a chief quality officer or chief safety officer is put in place, with key responsibilities that include the education of health system staff in how to use process improvement methods and tools that will support the organization's process improvement efforts. Hospital departments frequently appoint physician and nursing quality champions in this phase, ushering in the next phase of quality through personnel development. Designed to provide sustainable leadership, health system quality and safety leaders become the responsible agents who are charged with evaluating the systematic deployment of quality tools at a local level while stimulating interdisciplinary teams to engage in improvement efforts that are measured and reported publicly. In this phase of maturity, defect rates range from one in ten thousand to one in one hundred thousand, and strong reinforcing structures are put in place that allow for identification of even small defects. In this quality-improvement phase, processes continue to be monitored to ensure that the improvements remain under statistical control.

The final level of maturity focuses on creating a structure that is inclusive of patients and families in new care design processes that are not only effective and efficient but also focus on the care experience itself, driving greater degrees of satisfaction for both health-care providers and care consumers. In this phase, new tools are created using novel resources such as the electronic health record to hardwire quality and safety improvements, making reporting of results more timely and accurate while also providing the ability to more deeply analyze data from the improvements that have been put in place. In this phase, defect rates can be as low as one defect per one hundred thousand care episodes to one defect in one million care episodes. When health-care providers, consumers, and administrators all align around a single structure such as this, high-value health-care services that promote a patient-centered approach that yields high quality outcomes and cost efficiency become sustainable over time.

Process. As health system quality efforts mature, there are new opportunities to deploy more sophisticated quality tools that reinforce their sustaining structures. As health-care quality leaders begin shaping the vision for higher degrees of quality and safety, they use a tool called the Change Acceleration Process (CAP), developed by the General Electric Corporation in their efforts to promote more rapid implementation of improvement projects.[117,118] Deploying a set of performance improvement tools, the GE solutions focus on people, process, and technology to learn from each rapid improvement cycle. Tools have also begun to be translated from other non-health-care industries such as the use of the Toyota Production System, which reinforces a systematic approach to focus on removing waste and inconsistency,[119] while even more sophisticated statistically focused improvement tools have been deployed by some systems that establish goals of producing six-sigma levels of quality, where fewer than 3.4 defects per million patient encounters can be seen. By focusing on tools and methods that address health-care process defects, care systems are now able to take longer and faster strides in their efforts to sustain process improvement gains while decreasing system complexity and costs.

One such health system, the Virginia Mason Medical Center in Seattle, Washington, has been recognized as a world leader in health-care transformation by embracing the improvement principles espoused by Toyota, sending its health-care quality leaders to Japan for annual training from the originators of the auto manufacturer's lean manufacturing processes.[120] Virginia Mason's commitment to designing processes that reduce waste from each of their care processes began in 2002, and the quality-improvement methods have translated into their ability to offer money-back warranties for some surgical procedures should defects arise during the course of evaluation and treatment.[121]

---

117 Bob Von Der Lin, HPT blog, accessed March 21, 2017, https://bvonderlinn.wordpress.com/2009/01/25/overview-of-ges-change-acceleration-process-cap/.

118 B. Becker, M. Huselid, and D. Ulrich, *The HR Scorecard; Linking People, Strategy, and Performance* (Boston: Harvard Business School Press, 2001).

119 J. K. Liker, *The Toyota Way: 14 Management Principles from the World's Greatest Manufacturer* (New York: McGraw-Hill, 2004).

120 "Center for Health Care Improvement Science," Virginia Mason Medical Center, Seattle, WA, accessed May 24, 2017, https://www.virginiamason.org/center-health-care-improvement-science.

121 "Virginia Mason Warranty for Hip and Knee Replacement Surgery," accessed March 21, 2017, https://www.virginiamason.org/Warra.

By specifying the desired health-consumer-focused value in the care processes offered, by formally mapping the care process to identify areas of opportunity, and by using waste-reducing process improvements, others such as Theda Care Health System in Appleton, Wisconsin, and Cincinnati Children's Hospital in Ohio have reinforced the utility of the lean process improvement models.

Just as Toyota helped improve health system performance by reducing waste from health-care delivery processes, other high-risk industries have been studied to help create models of care process improvement. The DuPont STOP (Safety Training Observation Program) has been modified from use in the high-risk chemical manufacturing industry and has been applied in health care to enhance safety systems. Efforts made by Memorial Health System in South Bend, Indiana, to reinforce the DuPont safety principles to redesign care processes for both health-care workers and health-care consumers generated many fewer safety incidents through their deployment and gave Memorial the recognition of being one of the safest health systems in the nation. Sentara Health System of Virginia Beach, Virginia, translated safety principles used in the nuclear power industry, such as more formal communication methods, to become a national best practice for their commitment to patient safety practices. Other high-risk safety principles were adopted by organizations such as Memorial Health System that were based on Dr. Thomas Krause's work with the aerospace industry, where active deployment of safety lessons that had been designed by NASA helped enhance health-care leadership safety practices.[122]

Outcomes. As both the public and payers began asking for quantitative results from health system quality and patient safety improvement efforts, several new communication channels began popping up as Internet resources that were designed to promote transparency in reporting health-care outcomes. Health systems began developing strategies to communicate their improvement efforts to their communities, and systems such as Middlesex Health System in Middletown, Connecticut, published one of the first community quality report cards in the nation to publicly highlight their quality and safety

---

122 Thomas R. Krause, *Leading with Safety* (Hoboken, NJ: Wiley & Sons, 2005).

efforts.[123] The publication was intended not only to help local residents better understand the results from the health system's quality efforts, but also to promote a discussion in the community regarding the personal relevance of the measures of quality being used. Government websites began to emerge, such as Hospital Compare from the Centers for Medicare and Medicaid Services,[124] that began collecting and reporting data regarding outcomes from care processes being deployed to treat common medical conditions, further engaging health-care consumers in discussions regarding the value of health care being delivered by specific institutions. Almost overnight, a cottage industry sprang forth to capture the demand being expressed by health-care consumers that they needed more and better information about health care to become activated participants in their own health-care experiences. Awards recognizing hospital and health system quality and patient safety efforts became commonplace, with methodologies that were frequently highly proprietary and with poorly communicated methodologies. Using a star ranking system or a "Top Health System" designation, companies began recognizing high-performing systems, leading to debate about the validity of methods employed to create these rankings. Some, such as Lindenauer and Bratzler, published results stating that hospitals engaged in both public reporting and pay for performance achieved greater improvements than those engaged solely in reporting, suggesting that financial incentives may help drive improvement efforts as an adjunct to simply reporting health-care outcomes.[125] Still others issued caution concerning the use of publicly reported measures to drive improvements given questions about the relevance of data being collected and reported.[126,127]

123 "Middlesex Hospital Quality & Compliance," accessed March 21, 2017, https://middlesex-hospital.org/middlesex-and-the-community/quality-and-compliance.

124 "Hospital Compare," accessed March 21, 2017, http://www.medicare.gov/hospitalcompare.

125 P. K. Lindenauer et al., "Public Reporting and Pay for Performance in Hospital Quality Improvement," *New England Journal of Medicine* 356, no. 5 (2007): 486–496.

126 J. M. Austin et al., "Fostering Transparency in Outcomes, Quality, Safety, and Costs," *Journal of the American Medical Association* 316, no. 16 (2016): 1661–1662.

127 R. A. Berenson and D. R. Kaye, "Grading a Physician's Value—The Misapplication of Performance Measurement," *New England Journal of Medicine* 369, no. 22 (2013): 2079–2081.

Underlying principles regarding methods to change provider behaviors have promoted transparency and reporting as being drivers for improvement, but disagreement still exists in how to best use data to enhance health-care practices. Writing in *JAMA* in 2008, Holmboe suggested that medical knowledge is certainly tied to health-care quality, but further study is needed to determine how best to incorporate knowledge expansion into practice patterns that ultimately improve patient care.[128] Supporting the very local nature of improvement science, the Institute for Healthcare Improvement's Don Berwick proposed that clinical outcomes improvement science is best applied at the local microsystem level of a health system community, where care can be best delivered "for the right patient at the right time all of the time."[129] Supporting Berwick's call for local microsystem improvements, Lee and colleagues studied the outcomes resulting from instituting programs to reduce variation that demonstrated benefit to physicians attempting to change their practice patterns.[130] Not only were clinical outcomes improved in Lee et al.'s review, but the overall total cost of care for certain conditions was reduced, leading the authors to suggest that physician behaviors could be modified if appropriate information was given to the provider during the care experience.

In 2003, the Institute of Medicine (IOM) published the third in a series of quality and safety improvement reports that identified ongoing issues in health-care value.[131] Stating that problems of health-care quality remained prevalent, the IOM cautioned that Americans risked becoming desensitized to quality and safety concerns, even as change and improvement were being pursued. In response, several organizations have continued to step forward to lead performance improvement efforts at scale, including the Institute for Healthcare

128 E. S. Holmboe et al., "Assessing Quality of Care—Knowledge Matters," *Journal of the American Medical Association* 299, no. 3 (2008): 338–340.

129 D. Berwick, *Institute for Healthcare Improvement. Idealized Design of Clinical Office Practice* (Boston: Institute for Healthcare Improvement, 2000).

130 V. S. Lee et al., "Implementation of a Value-Driven Outcomes Program to Identify High Variability in Clinical Costs and Outcomes and Association with Reduced Cost and Improved Quality," *Journal of the American Medical Association* 316, no. 10 (2016): 1061–1072.

131 Institute of Medicine, *Priority Areas for National Action. Transforming Health Care Quality* (Washington, DC: National Academies Press, 2003).

Improvement, whose programs have included national improvement efforts such as "Saving 100,000 Lives" and the "Five Million Lives Campaign," which were both aimed at identifying specific interventions to minimize the low-quality care experiences from the use of nonstandard approaches to care.[132] Other improvement efforts, such as the American Hospital Association's pioneering work through its Health Research & Educational Trust division, have shown great promise in helping improve quality and safety metrics through the Hospital Engagement Network (HEN) and Hospital Improvement Innovation Network (HIIN). These efforts have focused on implementation of high-value care practices at thousands of hospitals in the United States, saving tens of thousands of lives and reducing billions of dollars in health-care costs from federal budgets by promoting the deployment of standardized high-value care practices.[133] Issuing recommendations on how to proceed in the new millennium, the IOM suggested that a framework should be determined that would maximize the value of organizational improvements that embrace how hospitals can best coordinate treatment of chronic illness, create a focus on improving acute health-care practices, enhance preventive care strategies, and promote more effective care at the end of life.[134] They identified a list of priority areas for improvement that would most likely create the highest degree of impact on disability, mortality, and economic cost encompassing a broad range of individuals without regard to race, gender, ethnicity, or socioeconomic status.

A final opportunity for health-care systems to achieve accelerated improvements is through engagement of the entire community in developing health-care process improvement solutions. As consumers become more deeply engaged as invited members of quality and safety project teams, their values, reflecting the needs and wishes of an entire community, can be incorporated into the design of new health-care processes. An example of how health-care

---

132 Institute for Health Care Improvement website, accessed March 21, 2017, http://www.ihi.org/.
133 Health Research & Educational Trust website, accessed March 21, 2017, http://www.hret-hiin.org/.
134 *Future Directions for the National Healthcare Quality and Disparities Reports*, Institute of Medicine Report, Agency for Healthcare Research and Quality, accessed May 23, 2017, https://www.ahrq.gov/research/findings/final-reports/iomqrdrreport/index.html.

consumer preferences can be incorporated into care design comes from work done in West Bend, Wisconsin, when the new St. Joseph's Hospital was being planned. When Dr. John Reiling encouraged formation of a study group to ensure that the new facility would be designed using proven safety principles, the West Bend community embraced its role to assist in deployment of patient-focused facility design.[135] Another example comes from South Bend, Indiana, where Memorial Health System engaged IDEO, a global design company, to monitor patient and family movement through a cardiology care experience by taking snapshots of patients as they made stops at the admissions department, laboratory, radiology, and finally the cardiac catheterization laboratory and postprocedure recovery area.[136] Coupling information obtained by photographic images that directly visualized the actual care delivery processes with patient and family interviews made it clear that the initial heart hospital facility design was fraught with error in that community preferences had not been incorporated into the proposal. Using a deep dive process designed by its innovation team, Memorial developed a new heart hospital care model that reinforced an improved facility design that not only was more efficient in providing care, but was also tailored precisely to the needs of the community, focusing on better patient intake and promotion of support services such as healthy nutrition, medication education, and exercise programs.

Since health care remains an intensely personal experience, the health status of an individual or a population of patients is still defined by the effective caring relationships between those receiving care and those delivering it. The social compact that governs this relationship has come under great scrutiny of late, given the pressures of health-care finance reform policy, the call to measure the results from the "health-care transaction" through public reporting, and the strain caused from reduced access to some health-care providers and the diminishing amount of time being spent with health-care providers. Quality and safety, with the resultant perceptions about the health-care experience, are largely influenced by the bond formed between provider and

---

135 J. Reiling, *Safe by Design: Designing Safety in Health Care Facilities, Processes, and Culture* (Oakbrook Terrace, IL: Joint Commission Resources, 2007).

136 Newbold and Stover-Hopkins, *Wake Up and Smell the Innovation.*

consumer of care, making efforts to preserve and enhance that bond paramount in our way forward toward creating the world's best health-care delivery system. Regardless of the many policy changes that bring new definition every day to the way that health care is to be most efficiently delivered and reimbursed, the social compact that has been present for hundreds of years should be the last component of the health-care experience to be abandoned. Bringing health-care consumers and providers together to fulfill a common vision of improving health-care practices while preserving the "caring" component of the health-care experience should remain the focal point for all discussions about health-care financing that arise in state legislatures and on Capitol Hill.

Key Points to Master From Chapter 7

- Two seminal works were released by the Institute of Medicine in 1999 and 2001 that called into question the success of American health care's pursuit of excellence in quality and safety programming.
- Regarding health care's inability to innovate in a timely fashion and across a broad range of practitioners, Everett Rogers' study on farming methods demonstrated that human behavior transcends occupation. It is difficult to change one's practices, and the rate of change to adopt new methods is limited by one's position on the adoption curve.
- Five key stages of the Rogers model include:
  o Knowledge acquisition: exposure to new information
  o Persuasion: efforts made by others to promote change in practice
  o Decision: lengthy process to resolve conflicts and move forward
  o Implementation: design and deployment of a new approach
  o Confirmation: measurement and demonstration of success
- The Six Aims from the IOM to describe safe and high-quality care:
  o Safe
  o Timely
  o Effective
  o Efficient
  o Equitable
  o Patient-centered
- Defective learning theory practices that reduce likelihood of success:
  o Use of "Cargo Cult mentality" solutions
  o Creating "Fordlandia"
  o Defects with clarity of definitions and methods
  o Clinical dogmatism
- The Donabedian Model for improvement has three elements:
  o Structure: program construct (Quality Control, Quality Improvement, Quality Personnel Development, Quality through Innovation) and leadership (communicator, data user, searches for multiple inputs, experience building teams, focused on results).

o   Process: Tools to support change such as PDCA cycles, Change Acceleration Process, lean, six sigma, full one-day process workouts
o   Outcome: Use of data to tell the story of how the process created the result, using vibrant narrative and graphic representation.

Eight

THE ASCENT OF HEALTH INFORMATICS

At a different time in a galaxy far away, there existed a reality where the medical records department of a hospital was a physical plant housing handwritten or transcribed and typed records of a patient's progress during an inpatient stay. Information pertinent to the patient's outpatient experience was frequently held inside the practitioner's head, to be retrieved from the mental vault much like the recall of a person with photographic memory. In more formalized offices, the medical record consisted of file cards that contained one-line summaries of the day's patient visits, comprising only each patient's diagnosis and office interventions. In even more advanced offices, rows and rows of alphabetized medical records jackets were stacked neatly on shelves in a special room in the office from which records could be pulled for a physician office visit, and these "medical charts" served as the final resting spot for X-ray reports, laboratory test results, and insurance information. This arrangement sufficed in an era of medical paternalism, when patients deferred to solitary physician providers, imploring their doctors to act on their best behalf based on information that was more informally catalogued. Medical offices often needed to employ one or more full-time employees to manually file paper records and to stuff into office charts the additional reports that came from reference laboratories and ancillary hospital departments. Having access to personal health-care information was not widely valued by patients who found their own health care to be much too complex and scientific to comprehend. As the health-care provider–consumer relationship evolved, so too did the appearance of the medical record, the types of data it contained, how it was to be used, and the rules governing access to this private and protected information.

When the Health Insurance Portability and Accountability Act (HIPAA) was signed into law by President Clinton in 1996, Title I of the act protected workers and their families from loss of health insurance should the primary insured individual lose or change jobs.[137] A secondary component of the act was Title II, which called for establishment of national standards for electronic health transactions and created national identifiers for health-care providers, insurance companies, and employers. It is from the second component of the act that access to electronic health information has irreversibly changed, coming under greater control and scrutiny of the federal government.[138] HIPAA's Title II defined policies, procedures, and methods to protect individually identifiable health information and outlined civil and criminal penalties for violating the statute. In response to this new law, health-care institutions and practitioner offices began to formalize internal policies and procedures to become compliant with the law, thus changing the pace at which electronic health records would be deployed. It is a stretch to believe that HIPAA caused electronic medical records to come into existence, but the regulations under HIPAA did escalate the speed of their adoption and formalized the practices surrounding their use.

The use of electronic information resources has been in place since the development of the first personal computer (PC), but extensive use of electronic health information is only a relatively recent phenomenon. Using computerized resources began in academic medical centers primarily to support research and clinical activities, and widespread use of "minicomputers" as bedside adjuncts did not fully come into favor until the 1990s with the

---

137 B. K. Atchinson and D. M. Fox, "The Politics of the Health Insurance Portability and Accountability Act," *Health Affairs* 16, no. 3 (1997): 146–150.

138 "Administrative Simplification Overview/HIPAA," accessed March 23, 2017, www.cms.gov.

advent of the PC. Early efforts to access information to better care for patients using electronic diagnostic and therapeutic resources were often asynchronous, bulky, and slow. These resources were typically quite similar to printed resources but had the advantage of being able to be retrieved electronically instead of requiring a practitioner to access printed materials that quickly became outdated. In the 1980s, with lighter-weight personal computers leading the way, health-care treatment information became available for clinicians who were willing to carry computers to the bedside, where patient data needed to be hand-entered to yield the care suggestions that were regurgitated back to the provider. These systems, referred to as "luggables," were portable in name only, as they frequently weighed between twenty and thirty pounds and needed to be connected through wired portals.

One pioneer in the use of luggables was a clinical cardiologist, Dr. T. M. Brown ("The T. M. stands for treadmill," he would say to his patients), who carried a shoulder bag containing such a computer, demonstrating the intrinsic value of having a "peripheral brain" available to assist him in expanding the diagnostic possibilities for his patient's clinical complaints. Not only was the computer too heavy to carry for an entire day's hospital work, it also added several minutes to each patient's clinical encounter and generally provided the same differential diagnosis that Brown had originated himself. The point had been made, however, that additional resources, if provided in a timely fashion, could serve as a significant adjunct to some clinicians, helping them consider options that had not been clearly apparent. Other adjuncts to medical practices, such as "virtual information" that was made available as floppy discs and CDs, were being sold to providers to use in their offices to enhance diagnostic testing strategies and to provide general medical information that could be easily printed and distributed to patients and their families at the time of an office visit. These early pilot uses of computerized information seemed to lack a longer-term vision of how they might be used as a significant contributor to the care of a large population of patients with unique health-care needs.

With the growing emergence of a need for electronic health resources and management tools in the 1990s, several companies began to provide consulting services for health-care delivery systems that had tried initially to customize their electronic medical records processes. Initial solutions were designed to provide a more comprehensive view of a patient's hospital care plan while also providing access at multiple sites of service, ranging from hospitals to primary-care and specialist offices. These computer software support companies, such as McKesson-HBOC, Cerner, and Epic, became synonymous with "advanced care," as they promised a future where all information regarding a patient could be housed in a single place from which that information could be used by anyone with the appropriate security clearance. This longitudinal electronic medical record was viewed as a new communication channel that would save clinicians time while enhancing the clinical outcomes for thousands of patients. The financial efficiencies and improvement in health-care processes created by using computerized records were touted as the justification for a large initial cost outlay to purchase such new and wonderful technology, and many hospitals deferred calculating a specific return on investment, seeing the new computer era as the next step in their evolution as an integrated delivery network. Many health systems even used their prowess in information technology to their marketing advantage, suggesting that the implementation of electronic information tools distinguished them from their competitors. Evanston Northwestern Hospital, winner of the Davies Award in 2004 for innovation in information technology, was one of the earliest adopters of a comprehensive strategy regarding use of electronic medical records, being recognized as the first system-wide electronic record that captured both integrated ambulatory and inpatient data.

From a recent federal government infographic, the future direction of health information technology appears to be leading communities to greater use of electronic resources by both providers and consumers of care. In this survey of health-care consumers, two out of every three stated that they would consider switching physicians, shifting from an office that did not use electronic medical records to one that did have access to records through a secure Internet connection, despite the fact that many Americans still have reservations about the validity of information found on health websites.[139] Even with

---

139 *2011 Survey of Health Care Consumers in the United States. Key Findings, Strategic Implications* (Washington, DC: Deloitte Center for Health Solutions, 2011).

some expressing reluctance to fully embrace the treatment suggestions found on the Internet, 80 percent of adult Internet users have routinely accessed the Internet for information regarding specific diseases or treatment plans.[140] Pointing to improvements in health outcomes related to implementation of new electronic health information strategies, the Network for Excellence in Health Innovation (NEHI), a nonprofit, nonpartisan national health policy institute, supported the direction taken by federal legislation to use electronic health records to monitor and manage chronic illnesses using electronic provider visits, use provider-patient portals to enhance transfer of clinical information, and promote tools to assist in stronger adherence to medication management strategies.[141] The federal government hoped that consumers accessing the Internet for medical resources would be better informed consumers of health care and that this newly empowered group would help manage medical services utilization and actively help reduce the total cost of health care.

The stage had been set to introduce American health care to computerization, but what actually transpired over the next twenty years? Since the earliest days when electronic health records were targeted solely as data repositories for individual patients, health information technologies have provided ease of reporting of the lengthy list of quality and safety metrics that have been in demand by the federal and state government, private health insurers, and freestanding evaluators of health-care effectiveness and efficiency. Many of these evaluators provided initial rewards to health-care systems that provided data electronically and penalized others that couldn't submit in this fashion. As greater numbers of work process metrics were requested by payers, a new cottage industry was created to help health systems in reporting and demonstrating improvement in key areas to show how medical informatics could deliver additional value to those systems.

---

140 Susannah Fox, "The Social Life of Health Information, 2011," Pew Research Center, Internet, Science and Tech, May 2011, accessed March 23, 2017, www.pewinternet.org/2011/05/12/the-social-life-of-health-information-2011/.
141 The Network for Excellence in Health Innovation, accessed March 23, 2017, www.nehi.net.

One such organization, the Hospital Management Systems Society (HMSS), started with fewer than fifty industrial engineers who were interested in studying the benefits that could result from introducing hospital management engineering principles to enhance the quality of hospital work processes.[142] The organization charged itself to search for new methods and techniques that could create greater value of hospital services by streamlining administrative processes. From these early days of process improvement, the group proposed a new subsection called the Society for Computer Information Systems in 1972, but at this early date, it was felt that there was not a need for such a narrowly focused body. In response to greater numbers of new members coming from computer-science backgrounds, the organization changed its name in 1986 to HIMSS (including the *I* for "Information") to better recognize the new direction of the organization as a collection of information-technology experts. Today, the organization has expanded to more than fifty-two thousand members across hundreds of disciplines, and in 2013, the HIMSS annual conference drew nearly forty thousand attendees. Health information technology had arrived in force, and newly minted positions such as chief information officer (CIO) and chief medical information officer (CMIO) came to join health system senior leadership teams that were attempting to harness the power of health system investments of millions of dollars in information technology.

When asked about today's infatuation with information technology, one CMIO described the great promise of electronic health records by pointing to the many ways in which the health-care delivery system had morphed from a primitive system of paper records that could not be used for improvement efforts in any meaningful way to the state in which we find them today. Now electronically gathered, painstakingly collated, dissected into data marts residing in organizational data warehouses, capable of being accessed by clinicians and researchers to generate new knowledge, today's electronic health resources have been able to document improvements in the practice of medicine. This same information systems executive also cited the many ways that health-care

---

142 "History of the Healthcare Information and Management Systems Society," accessed March 23, 2017, www.himss.org/about/history.

consumers are now better engaged in accessing their own health information and how these consumers are becoming more active participants in their own care experience due to availability of clinical information that helps guide their decisions.

To more fully capture the impact from the ascent of the electronic health record, it is necessary to evaluate the impact of the benefits and challenges that have resulted from the introduction of this new engine of change.

- **Benefits.** The use of electronic data has produced significant benefits, beginning with the ability to capture data and radiographic images that can be stored in a single location so that clinicians can query them for a variety of uses. These records remove the hurdle of translating illegible handwritten entries, assist in medication reconciliation to identify errors in medicines taken by patients, and reduce the threat of lost medical records since they could be accessed at any location that connects to the health system's mainframe. These systems also make billing systems more efficient: electronic medical records drive more accurate capture of appropriate billing codes that can be better used when assessing health system performance. With information-technology resources now merging clinical and financial data, the true cost of care for medical illnesses and surgical procedures can be better quantitated, and system improvement efforts quantified. While many clinicians disparaged electronic medical records as being relevant only to hospital environments, the use of these new charting methods has proved essential to doctor's office practices across the country.

    A new field of applied informatics takes a wide array of information, merges key elements, and allows for conclusions to be drawn that shed light on the advisability of continuing historic care practices or shifting care strategies to incorporate innovative solutions that would otherwise only be recognized through lengthy and costly medical studies that require the use of complex statistical methods. With thousands of hospital admissions and millions of data entry points made available each year, most health systems that use electronic health information strategies can quickly determine the benefit-risk balance of introducing new care techniques at larger scale, or assess the consequences of performing or withholding certain tests and treatments on the clinical outcomes of patients. This decision-making process, based on what has been labeled "big data," allows an organization's data scientists to assess hundreds of what-if scenarios where improvement hypotheses can be constructed and tested using enormous amounts of data, and recommendations for care improvements can be provided to clinicians to assist in their evaluation of existing care practices.

The interest in providing "just-in-time information" to clinicians continues, evolving from its early days when ease of access was a significant challenge. Some clinicians had grown frustrated with a process where they needed to toggle away from a patient's clinical record to access the Internet for resources that were needed to make decisions at the bedside. This nonlinear or asynchronous access to information was likened by one medical informaticist to the winter Olympic sport of the biathlon, where athletes quickly travel on cross-country skis for long periods, only to have their momentum stopped when they need to hoist their rifle, shoot accurately at several targets, and then get back on their skis. In the medical world, long periods of time spent accessing a patient's medical record, entering data from a clinical encounter, and proffering a medical diagnosis could be interrupted by a need to stop to access the medical literature to assist in finalizing an approach to patient care. The advent of clinical decision support (CDS) has afforded clinicians the opportunity of more directly accessing information using an in-line information flow, with relevant clinical information presented to them much like the way that a freeway on-ramp allows for smooth flow of traffic. Data can be presented as needed to evaluate a patient or used to broaden a list of diagnostic and treatment approaches seamlessly at the point of care, thereby reducing interruptions found in previous efforts to access and use medical information and guaranteeing greater efficiency in care delivery.

Data presented to clinicians can also be harnessed for use in clinical research, and studies of human behavior can provide a better understanding of how change models work to alter a clinician's approach to old problems using newly deployed solutions. One such example of using electronic medical record data to create a new pattern of care stemmed from research conducted by Dr. Michael Rakotz at NorthShore University HealthSystem in Evanston, Illinois. As a family physician and a member of the first quality fellowship class that was designed to empower young physicians to more actively engage in producing system changes to promote higher quality and patient safety in care delivery, Rakotz made an observation about the lack of control in patients with high blood pressure. Deploying improvement techniques that addressed key defects in standard patient-care approaches that resulted in many patients not being recognized as having high blood pressure, Rakotz identified these patients using thousands of information points from multiple sites of service. By identifying patients who had not been previously diagnosed with high blood pressure and encouraging them to visit a medical office for validation of their blood-pressure readings, Rakotz helped patients who were suffering from a silent killer seek improved care. Working with newly developed mathematical algorithms, he was able to demonstrate that applied informatics could be used to identify the existing diagnosis and treatment gaps found in traditional care practices. Completing the improvement cycle he outlined, the patients who had been identified to be at risk received special attention to search for treatable causes for their elevations in blood pressure. When treated with high-blood-pressure medication, their blood pressures normalized, saving many lives from the ravages of cardiovascular complications such as stroke and heart attack.[143,144]

---

143 B. Coons, February 26, 2015, accessed March 23, 2017, http://blog.nm.org/home/northwestern-medicines-dr-rakotz-recognized-as-hypertension-control-champion.

144 J. DeGaspari, "The 2013 Healthcare Informatics Innovator Awards: First Place Winner: NorthShore University HealthSystem," *Healthcare Informatics: Healthcare IT Leadership, Vision, and Strategy.*

An extension of the use of big data to solve problems is in the development of the new field of predictive analytics. If one can use data from electronic health records to point the way toward improvement in diagnosis and treatment of existing conditions, imagine the benefit that could be obtained if one could actually *predict* the onset of disease or the likelihood that a condition might produce death or grave disability. Could medical records data, when appropriately extracted, collated, and analyzed, identify people who might be at risk of such future complications, and could the arc of these complications be altered, thereby promoting a better health status? When large volumes of data are used to better understand the natural history of a disease, conclusions can be drawn regarding the future state of that disease within a defined degree of comfort. Such is the case when looking at the projected mortality for an individual patient with a disease who has been compared to large numbers of patients with similar characteristics. Providing that information to a patient and family could assist treatment teams in their work with those families to provide more evolved person-focused medical-care interventions. Capturing individual patient preferences and values-driven preferences for care allows clinical teams to offer care strategies that are more in keeping with patient preferences as data are shared with patients and families. An example of the utility of information sharing can be seen when clinicians hold conversations with patients about palliative-care treatment strategies that recognize and respect the wishes of a person who is making an advanced-care planning decision. Similarly, if large data sets support the likelihood that a patient might fail in a home setting but succeed in an institutionalized setting, then future care gaps with disabling consequences could be avoided using data to discuss these differences.

Another benefit of having electronic clinical information available in large data sets is research being done to try to harness the power of supercomputing.[145] IBM's Watson, named for the first CEO

145 "Putting Watson to Work: Watson in Healthcare," IBM, accessed March 23, 2017, https://www.ibm.com/watson/health/value-based-care/?lnk=mpr_buwh.

of International Business Machines, has been used by a number of health systems to more comprehensively assess patient treatment plans based on the most current medical literature. Although more research is needed to adapt supercomputers to the daily care for patients, the future appears bright for bridging the human characteristics of care decision-making with the vast array of knowledge that can be gleaned from such computational devices.

Still other organizations are using atypical sources of data to research potential solutions for thorny health-care decisions, such as treatment for genetically associated diseases. Called "personalized medicine," databases are created from merging a wide array of patient data from clinical encounters, family history archives, and genetic snapshots called genomes. Strategies arising from the use of such databases help identify key markers in a patient's personal health information, and they can be used to customize treatment plans such as the use of tailored antibiotics for serious infections or gene-driven care for more effective cancer treatments. Called pharmacogenomics, this approach merges information from a variety of sources and gauges the likelihood of success of a highly personalized treatment option when compared to the alternatives. From a recent survey of health professionals, about a third of respondents felt that their hospitals would be using whole-genome sequencing for patients with unknown diseases within the next five years.[146] With innovations in genetic sequence technology, the cost to sequence a human genome has plummeted, and it is expected that more efficient cancer treatment strategies will result from a better understanding of a person's clinical and genomic data, captured in a clinical analytics database.[147]

146 E. J. Topol, "The Era of Individualized Medicine," *FutureScan 2015*, American College of Healthcare Executives and the Society for Healthcare Strategy & Market Development (Chicago: Health Administration Press).

147 E. J. Topol, *The Creative Destruction of Medicine* (New York: Basic Books, 2012).

Finally, the benefits of advanced computing can be seen as health-care consumers become more deeply involved in directing the care plans being prescribed for them. Playing the role of "orchestra conductors," health-care consumers now want to have input into the final musical score of their health-care planning, and electronic health information portals have begun to give health-care consumers greater power in fulfilling this promise. Starting with electronic data repositories where patients could check their test results, patient portals quickly evolved to a place where patients can ask questions of their providers and receive replies asynchronously to help gain a better understanding of their medical conditions, assess next steps in a treatment plan, and provide feedback to their clinicians about the effectiveness of a prescribed medical treatment. Electronic communication channels with tertiary health system subspecialists using telemedicine channels have allowed patients to remain at home in front of their computer to interact with remote specialists hundreds of miles away to streamline their clinical encounters. Some health systems have built facilities to promote examination by specialists using a computer interface, supplemented by special examination equipment modified for use by patients during such examinations. Still other "telehealth" solutions have arisen at employer work sites to reduce the time spent away from work when an employee is scheduled to see a clinician in a remote office setting. By connecting directly through a computer interface, health-care consumers can access medical assistance without having to leave the work site, thereby saving time and lost productivity.

Two additional self-directed care efforts promoted through information technology are the use of biowearable devices to deliver health information and the use of health-care blogging to secure medical information. Just as with other cottage industries that have arisen around institutional electronic health information, companies have sprung forward with a variety of devices designed to measure heart rate, blood pressure, body weight, and other biometric data such as electrocardiographic tracings, medication level monitoring, and changes in skin salt content.[148] As newer methods evolve, health-care consumers will continue to access them as they express their demand for control of their own medical information. Serving as advisors or navigators, disease-specific blogs have been launched for consumers to connect with one another as they seek advice and solutions to diagnostic challenges, assess the perceived value of treatment and complications, and select care providers for children or elderly parents.

How health-care consumers and providers use electronic health information appears to be consistent with the initial purpose set forth when the Internet was created: "to serve as a world-wide broadcasting capability, a mechanism for information dissemination, and a medium for collaboration and interaction between individuals and their computers without regard for geographic location."[149] Without electronic medical records, highly valuable patient portals that stimulate asynchronous communication between providers and care consumers could not exist, and ancient communication strategies such as waiting for telephonic responses would still exist today.

- **_Challenges._** With so many benefits seen from having access to electronic medical resources, diagnostic strategies, and enhanced treatment planning, it is sometimes difficult to remember that there also exist some limitations and challenges inherent in today's use of electronic health strategies. For some people, the use of electronic health records has created new challenges that have made the health-care experience less rewarding, and the administrative and time challenges found in changing health-care delivery practices in the computer age have produced a great deal of discomfort for those delivering care, particularly for those who began providing care in the precomputerized health-record age. Three main challenges have arisen from the ascent of the electronic health record: accuracy of health information

---

148 Daniel Kraft, Singularity University, accessed May 3, 2017, https://su.org/faculty-speakers/daniel-kraft/.

149 B. M. Leiner et al., "Brief History of the Internet," *The Internet Society*, accessed March 23, 2017, http://internetsociety.org.

and its maintenance by health-care providers functioning as data-entry clerks, the financial implications of hardware and software and maintenance thereof, and the erosion of the relationship between caregiver and care consumer, often categorizing the computer as "the third person in the room."

As with any other computer system, the accuracy of information that comes from the electronic health record is directly related to the accuracy of information put into the device. Errors of data entry can be created when persons receiving care misinterpret questions asked of them, when technical terms are not understood, when persons are disabled secondary to the medical injury that has befallen them, or when data entry is rushed, leading to what has been called "fat fingering errors." All of these defects can lead to errors of omission of vital information or errors of commission where information has been entered that does not accurately describe a patient's clinical condition or medical history. One such example is in the regulation to enter information describing a person's race, ethnicity, and language (REAL) data into a medical record for purposes of enhancing community health efforts. A personal friend and former colleague who immigrated to the United States from Argentina delivered three children in this country. One child carried the designation "Caucasian," mainly because his mother is a redheaded, fair-skinned South American who was perceived by a medical-records clerk to be "American"; one child was designated "Latino," since her parents spoke Spanish; and one was labeled "unknown." All three suffered from an error of omission, since the admitting clerk failed to ask the expectant mother about her actual REAL data. This data-entry error problem is significant and leads to many inappropriate conclusions regarding vital information, such as whether a person would like to have full resuscitation measures in the event that his or her heart were to stop or what exact medications a person is known to be allergic to. An informatics phrase, "garbage in, garbage out," has been created to describe such errors and the lack of ability to draw cogent conclusions. Although some quality checks exist, such as algorithms that identify extremely inaccurate data entries such as weights that dramatically change by more than 10 percent between entries, erroneous data can still be found in electronic medical records.

A second challenge or shortcoming of electronic health record system deployment is tied to the financial costs of implementing such systems. To promote the use of electronic health records for reporting and billing purposes, the federal government created a series of financial rewards for health systems that certify their adherence to certain industry standards needed to submit data electronically. Called Meaningful Use for Certified Health Record Technology, the rewards were based on three phases of documentation: the first in 2011 with demonstration of data capture and sharing expertise, a phase in 2014 to document advanced clinical process documentation, and a final phase in 2016 that certified the improvements in clinical outcomes.[150] Eligible hospitals were able to qualify for millions of dollars for attesting to their adherence to key certification demonstrations, and the rewards provided helped offset the initial investment the hospitals needed to make if they had not previously introduced electronic health records. Reaching an investment total of millions of dollars in hardware and software costs, with large departments of computer scientists adding additional layers of personnel costs, coupled with health information technology vendors' charges for system maintenance and development, the implementation and maintenance costs for electronic health records are a significant operating expense for most health systems. Many health systems began to wonder whether a return on investment (ROI) could ever be realized, and many more were skeptical that the data would ever become available to allow documentation of a favorable ROI, since a number of benefits remain present in a system that cannot be accurately estimated. With growing

150 "EHR Incentives and Certification," HealthIT.gov, accessed March 23, 2017, https://www.healthit.gov/providers-professionals/meaningful-use-definition-objectives.

consumer demands for access to electronic health information portals and to a portable medical record that would serve many health-care providers, some institutions see information technology as one reason that they need external access to capital, even fueling merger and acquisition discussions aimed at salvaging an organization's ability to continue operations.

The final challenge encountered from introduction of electronic health information systems is the change in the relationship between health-care provider and health-care consumer. What had at one time been a very personal face-to-face interview and examination was altered, as the introduction of an electronic interface began to be seen as an interference and distractor. Electronic health records were designed to promote greater degrees of communication, but many providers found that they were becoming so busy as data-entry clerks that the time needed to pursue a patient's medical concerns was being eroded. Some providers described the computer as "the patient" and the patient as "the bystander," reflecting the overblown importance given to the mechanical third person in the room. Adoption of the new device and the new information-recording processes appear to be somewhat age-dependent: older providers seem less likely to embrace computer-generated records, and this group often underappreciates the benefits that come with use of the electronic record. Some patients have expressed dissatisfaction with a computerized encounter, stating that they feel that the care provider is not fully present in the room with them and may appear distracted by the need to interact with the computer.

Some systems began giving guidance to their providers on where to locate the computer so that the patient and the provider might jointly communicate about the information being entered, with the computer occupying a shared space between them. Other systems encourage note-taking by providers with completion of the data-entry portion at a later time when the patient is no longer present. Still other systems have embraced the use of "scribes" whose job it is to enter data into the system as the provider and patient are more directly engaged in a traditional health-care encounter. While developing strategies to better integrate the electronic health record into the flow of a patient visit, most systems have asked tolerance from their providers and consumers of care until greater familiarity with electronic record keeping can be demonstrated, hopefully leading to greater benefits realized in health outcomes.

One conclusion that can clearly be drawn from this great social and technological experiment is that the rules of engagement remain in flux. As innovative efforts that are being pursued by health systems across the country yield favorable changes in work processes, this discovery will likely help define the many new roles and benefits for health information technology. One can only hope that the challenges needing to be addressed can be successfully overcome, maintaining at least a vestige of the health-care provider–consumer social compact that has been placed under duress. Only by doing so will the provider-patient bond be strengthened, helping to create greater satisfaction in both parties with improvement in the resultant clinical health care outcomes while promoting more fulfilling experiences of care that this stronger bond will generate.

Key Points to Master From Chapter 8

- The Health Insurance Portability and Accountability Act (HIPAA) of 1996 provided for protection of workers and their families from loss of health insurance should the primary insured individual lose or change jobs. A secondary component of the Act called for establishment of national standards for electronic health transactions and created national identifiers for health care providers, insurance companies, and employers.
- The 1980's and 1990's saw an explosion of computer support services and software companies that hoped to improve communication between all parties involved in the care experience, make care more effective, deliver on financial efficiencies, and distinguish health systems from their competitors.
- The Hospital Information Management Systems Society grew from a fledgling group with little focus on computing to a 50,000-member society that helped launch new executive health care careers such as the CIO and the CMIO.
- Multiple benefits have already been seen from health information technology including the use of electronic health information to support health care research, capturing electronic health information to support financial and clinical improvements, creating "what if" scenarios that provide useful clinical decision support, supercomputing and machine learning to expand information access at the point of service, fostering "personalized medicine" solutions, supporting consumer-directed care using patient portals to their health information, and stimulating remote access to care via telemedicine.
- Despite the benefits of electronic health information, several challenges remain, including the development of processes to collate, store, retrieve, and maintain information, the financial impact on health systems to purchase and maintain expanding health information departments, and the psychological impact on the consumer-provider bond from having a "third person in the room".

Nine

The Employer's Role in Health Insurance

A s the highly partisan debate about the future of American health-care financing options continues on Capitol Hill, it is important to understand the unique funding options for a significant protected class of insured individuals who are being covered through employer health plans. Nearly half of all Americans are provided employer-based health insurance coverage, and this percentage has decreased slightly from 2008, when 49.2 percent received coverage at work to 44.5 percent participating in employer-based plans in 2012[151]. Although some employers are beginning to assess the impact from the Affordable Care Act, no significant disruption of the employer insurance marketplace has yet been noted as a result of the policy changes that occurred in 2010. One of the great challenges faced by employers is how to continue providing health-care coverage for employees while maintaining financial margins in a global economy that has produced slow economic growth in the 1–2 percent per year range in the United States.[152] Health insurance coverage is one of the most sought-after benefits by employees, and firms are often

---

151 E. Mendes, "Fewer Americans Getting Health Insurance from Employers," *Gallup-Healthways Well-Being Index*, February 22, 2013, accessed March 27, 2017.

152 J. Ferreira, "United States GDP Growth Rate," *Trading Economics*, April 28, 2017, accessed May 17, 2017, http://www.tradingeconomics.com/united-states/gdp-growth.

finding themselves competing in the employee marketplace not just on wage and salary comparisons but on overall benefit packages that include medical, vision, and dental insurance. The grim reality for employers is that there has been a steady rise of 3–4 percent per year for premiums that has outpaced the overall growth of the American economy.[153] Before exploring what employers have done to offset the impact of rising premium costs that have impacted 90 percent of American businesses, some explanation is necessary for how employers first became engaged in providing health insurance as a benefit to employees.

American businesses began experimenting with provision of health insurance benefits as early as the 1920s and 1930s as a means of stabilizing the employee pools by reducing workforce losses tied to worker injury and illness and its deleterious effect on productivity.[154] It wasn't until World War II that a standard set of benefits was beginning to be offered to American workers. This standard package of insurance benefits arose largely because of the impact of federal wage freezes that occurred during a time when most of the country's economic engines were focused on the means of production of war-related goods and services. To retain excellent workers, private businesses began to add health insurance coverage as a perquisite for employees who were in short supply and high demand. These benefits required little administrative overhead and offered an additional benefit to employers in that they could also claim these benefit contributions as financial deductions to lower their corporate income taxes.[155]

Today, employer-provided health insurance brings more than just a degree of certainty to businesses in their efforts to reduce employee absenteeism, and it has become one of the major benefits required by many workers in an era

153 *Kaiser/HRET Survey of Employer Sponsored Health Benefits, 1999–2015*, released September 14, 2016, accessed March 27, 2017, http://kff.org/health-costs/report/2016-employer-health-benefits-survey/.

154 K. McDonnell, "History of Health Insurance Benefits," *Employee Benefit Research Institute*, March 2002, accessed May 17, 2017, https://www.ebri.org/publications/facts/index.cfm?fa=0302fact.

155 M. Roizen, *Sharecare, Inc.*, accessed March 27, 2017, https://www.sharecare.com/health/health-insurance/employer-sponsored-health-insurance.

where significant increases in the overall costs of health-care services have produced a great deal of risk aversion in employees. To put this benefit trend in perspective, over the past ten years, inflation has increased by 9 percent, workers' wages have increased slightly more at 10 percent, but health insurance premiums have increased by nearly three times these rates.[156] Since the percentage share of overall health insurance premium increases shouldered by workers has increased by 78 percent over this period, the impact of rising health-care costs has been quite significant in raising health insurance premium costs as well, preventing many employees from purchasing insurance on the open market as a simple out-of-pocket expense.[157]

Several federal health policies have impacted the insurance markets for employer-based plans dating back to 1965 when the Consolidated Omnibus Budget Reconciliation Act (COBRA) was passed to offer a degree of financial security to those employees who had suffered through a period of coverage loss when they left an employer because of relocation, termination, or global reductions in workforce.[158] COBRA provided continuation of coverage for employees departing a workplace but who wished to continue access to health-care coverage. Following discharge from an employer, a person would be allowed to pay the full cost of health premiums out of pocket to maintain coverage for a defined period of time using a COBRA administrative intermediary. This plan, while more expensive than a traditional employer-based health insurance plan where employer and employee share in insurance premiums, at least provided an avenue to continue health insurance without interruption. For many employees suffering through periods of high unemployment, there was some security in knowing that health-care coverage was assured, reducing the significant personal financial impact from serious illness or injury.

A second and equally important set of regulations came under the Employee Retirement Income Security Act (ERISA) of 1974, which defined

---

156 *Kaiser/HRET Survey of Employer Sponsored Health Benefits, 1999–2015*, accessed April 3, 2017.

157 Ibid.

158 The United States Department of Labor, *The Consolidated Omnibus Budget Reconciliation Act*, accessed May 17, 2017, https://www.dol.gov/general/topic/health-plans/cobra..

the documentation required by employers that chose to direct the administration of health benefits provided in their own work site.[159] ERISA regulations typically require employers to outline and disclose a variety of elements of such a plan, including the benefit design considerations; the fiduciary roles of the employer; how benefits will be fairly applied, including a process to resolve employee grievances related to benefit denials; an outline of the civil enforcement of plans as defined, including the legal remedies in cases of disagreement between worker and employer; and in which cases the plans are able to be administered under federal regulation rather than state laws. Specifically, if an employer chooses to create and maintain a self-insured plan and can meet the legal tests that define such a plan under ERISA statutes, the employer is offered great flexibility from state laws that mandate specific standard insurance coverage benefits for certain conditions or illnesses. In simple terms, if a firm offers coverage to its employees and spreads risk to include the entire population of workers, such a plan is deemed to be exempt from state insurance regulation. This preemption applies to decisions affecting how benefits are utilized and to the credentialing and certification of a provider network dictating the health-care providers being offered, and provides an exemption from being enjoined in medical malpractice claims as long as the benefits outlined in summary documents have been fairly applied by the business. Employers can choose to self-fund the plan and hold stop-loss insurance to prevent catastrophic medical claims that might bankrupt an employer-based plan that is self-funded, giving comfort to employees that their employer will have the financing to continuously provide benefits for all employees falling under coverage provisions.

Since ERISA-exempted, employer-based insurance is presented as a benefit to employees who participate in a health insurance plan, the employer can adjust benefit coverage and pricing much like traditional commercial insurers, but without stringent oversight by the state insurance commissioner. The trends and benefits changes seen in these specialized plans that have been implemented over the past several years have all come under the auspices

159 L. Wolfe, "What Is ERISA and What Does It Cover?," *the balance*, March 7, 2017, accessed May 17, 2017, https://www.thebalance.com/what-is-erisa-law-3515060.

of ERISA law, where employees are provided certain benefits at the time of their initial hire coupled with a defined premium-sharing structure that shelters employees from the true costs of health care.[160] Much research has been done on the benefits provided by employers and the impact on utilization of services.[161,162] Similarly, the proportion of costs shared between employer and employee and the trends in health plan design have been analyzed by a variety of research organizations, but the Kaiser Family Foundation (KFF), working in conjunction with the American Hospital Association's Health Research and Educational Trust (HRET), has yielded the most prominent longitudinal research on these delicate employment relationships, the latest of which was published in the fall of 2016.[163] The Kaiser/HRET Survey has provided a trend analysis that helps clarify some of the issues found in policy proposals being debated nationally. The following data and trends have been excerpted from the most recent Kaiser Family Foundation release on employer benefit coverage:

- *Sources for health insurance coverage.* As mentioned previously, approximately 44.5 percent of Americans receive health insurance benefits through their work, and this has declined by about 5 percent since 2008. The declines seen in employer-based coverage between 2008 and 2012 were largely due to both a spiraling increase in cost to provide insurance to employees secondary to medical inflation and changes in utilization, coupled with a rise in the unemployment rate. To retain some form of health insurance coverage, some

---

160 "Self-Insured Health Plans for Beginners," *Coastal Management Services*, 2011, accessed May 17, 2017, https://www.coastalmgmt.com/ppt/SIIA-Presentation.pdf.

161 J. L. Herman, "Costs and Benefits of Providing Transition-Related Health Care Coverage in Employee Health Benefits Plans," The Williams Institute, September 2013, accessed May 5, 2017, http://williamsinstitute.law.ucla.edu/wp-content/uploads/Herman-Cost-Benefit-of-Trans-Health-Benefits-Sept-2013.pdf.

162 B. Jackson, T. Gibson, and J. Staeheli, "Hospice Benefits and Utilization in the Large Employer Market," US Department of Health & Human Services, March 1, 2000, accessed May 7, 2017, https://aspe.hhs.gov/basic-report/hospice-benefits-and-utilization-large-employer-market.

163 *Kaiser/HRET Survey of Employer-Sponsored Health Benefits, 1999–2015*, accessed April 3, 2017.

underemployed Americans qualify for government health insurance plans such as Medicaid if they fall below the sliding poverty threshold, Medicare for the growing population of elderly baby boomers, or coverage provided under veteran's or military benefits. Summarizing all classes of government-provided health-care coverage, there was a 2.3 percent increase in individuals accessing benefits from federal and state sources between 2008 and 2012. For those who lost coverage when employers were driven out of the market due to spiking premium costs, about 17 percent of previously insured employees purchased insurance directly from the marketplace, an increase of approximately 2 percent in just five years. As a nation, the percentage of uninsured Americans remained flat at 11.1–11.5 percent, but since the country's population was rising, the absolute number of citizens without insurance continued to grow during this period. This growing pool of uninsured Americans creates a significant potential financial hazard for hospitals that do not have the ability to limit care to patients seeking treatment in emergency departments, given legislation that prevents patients from being turned away.[164] Not yet able to be measured is the impact on employers of certain provisions in the Patient Protection and Affordable Care Act, namely its requirement that employers with more than twenty employees provide health insurance or face the prospect of paying financial penalties for not doing so.

• ***Trends in benefit design and administration.*** Changes have also been seen in the plan designs provided by employers where less-rich plan benefit designs have been put in place as a means of continuing some degree of coverage for employees while allowing the business to maintain financial solvency. The largest coverage declines have been seen in plan designs using provider gatekeepers such as health maintenance organizations (HMOs), given employee dissatisfaction with such plans.

---

164 *Emergency Medical Treatment & Labor Act (EMTALA)*, Centers for Medicare and Medicaid Services, accessed May 17, 2017, https://www.cms.gov/Regulations-and-Guidance/Legislation/EMTALA/index.html.

Some employees seek to have greater choice of health-care providers and value the freedom to see their preferred providers despite costs being shifted to them in the form of higher copayments and coinsurance. HMO enrollment has dropped from approximately 20 percent of all employees in 2008 to less than 14 percent in 2015. Conventional indemnity designs have virtually disappeared due to their overall corporate cost, as healthier people have opted for less-rich benefit plans at lower monthly premium costs, leaving behind a risk pool of unhealthy individuals whose clinical conditions skew rates upward for everyone wishing to continue traditional insurance. Most employers continue to offer preferred provider organizations (PPOs) as a means of providing some degree of choice of provider network to employees while limiting access to a known provider panel that has been evaluated for cost and quality of care. The percentage of PPO enrollment in employer-based plans has remained stable in the 55–60 percent range for years, but in 2015, there seemed to be a shift to higher-deductible health plans, which will be discussed in the section below.

• *Trends in premium cost sharing.* One approach taken by many employers has been to shift some of the premium cost increases back to their employees. Still somewhat sheltering employees from the true costs of health insurance, employers are continuing efforts to educate their workers about the actual total cost of health insurance and the percentage being taken from their paychecks to provide insurance funding as part of a comprehensive benefits package. In 2015, employers paid 83 percent of the overall premium costs, while employees paid 17 percent. This ratio held for individual coverage; slightly greater amounts were being paid by employees enrolling their entire families in employer-based coverage. For smaller firms, the impact of providing family coverage is considerably greater, and employees of smaller companies bear approximately one-third of the premium costs for full family coverage.

Some employers have attempted to identify preventable health-care expenses by introducing health risk appraisals (HRAs), which are designed to recognize at-risk individuals who then enroll in an employer-based program designed to reduce future health-care costs.[165] In 2016, 59 percent of firms with at least two hundred employees offered or required an HRA, and 32 percent of firms provided a financial incentive such as a gift card or discounted health club memberships for employees completing the HRA. One such example is a small manufacturing company in central Iowa that had historically provided full coverage for traditional indemnity health insurance until the company's financial margins became squeezed to near zero. Looking for ways to limit growth of some individual expense line items, the firm shifted to a PPO plan with significant cost shifting for employees who chose to use care providers who were not in their preferred provider network. In addition, a health promotion strategy was initiated that included the use of HRAs to identify persons at risk for medical issues that had not been previously identified. Due to some suspicion on the part of employees that the HRA would be used to limit employment should a reduction of force become necessary, only 6 percent of employees chose to complete the health risk appraisal despite the firm's Human Resources Department assurances that the data would not be reported back to the company except in aggregate form. When one employee who had completed the HRA was found to be at substantial risk for colon cancer and had a colonoscopy performed that identified a precancerous condition, most employees began to see the benefit of what the firm was supporting. The following enrollment period, 95 percent of employees participated in the HRA process.

One additional aspect of risk appraisals is their ability to identify a need for worksite health promotion programs that can be customized to the company based on the aggregate HRA information. Such information promotes wellness and disease prevention and includes

---

165 V. J. Schoenbach, E. H. Wagner, and W. L. Beery, "Health Risk Appraisal: Review of Evidence for Effectiveness," *HSR: Health Services Research* 22, no. 4 (1987): 553–580.

programming targeted to reduce smoking, promote exercise, reduce stress, adjust eating behaviors to reduce cardiovascular disease, and modify risk factors that accompany chronic diseases such as diabetes, high blood pressure, and arthritis.

One significant trend in employee cost sharing has been the adoption of employer-based insurance coverage known as high-deductible health plans (HDHPs).[166] The fastest-growing type of employer-based coverage, HDHPs are frequently accompanied by health savings accounts (HSAs), which work like traditional savings plans for future health-care expenses and are fully portable from employer to employer.[167] The combination of HDHPs and HSAs allows employees to purchase health insurance coverage at lower premium costs. There is the potential, however, for greater out-of-pocket costs since the employee must first satisfy higher individual and family deductibles before coverage is paid by the company. For young and relatively healthy individuals, HDHPs reduce the amount withheld from each paycheck for health insurance premiums when there is little likelihood of need for coverage. The employee can then place those same pretax dollars into an HSA that can be used when illness or injury produces medical expenses at a later date. If an employee does not need those funds to satisfy out-of-pocket deductible expenses in a given year, those funds remain in the HSA and gain interest over time. As will be discussed in the discussion regarding replacement of the Affordable Care Act, some believe that HDHPs will be the norm for most workers and overall deductibles will increase for all service coverage, with one estimate of these increases being as much as a $1550 per person per year.[168]

---

166 G. E. Miller, "What Is a High Deductible Health Plan (HDHP)?," *20 something finance*, January 7, 2017, accessed May 15, 2017, https://20somethingfinance.com/what-is-a-high-deductible-health-plan-hdhp/.

167 "Health Savings Accounts (HSAs)," IRS Publication 969, accessed May 17, 2017, https://www.irs.gov/publications/p969/ar02.html#en_US_2016_publink1000204020.

168 D. Altman, "Why Deductibles Would Rise Under the GOP Health Care Plan," *Henry K. Kaiser Family Foundation* (blog), March 22, 2017, accessed March 27, 2017, Kff.org/health-reform/perspective.

- ***Special health premium issues.*** Employers may modify health insurance premiums paid by employees based on demonstration of healthy behaviors, and they can reward certain improvements in health status that lead to a reduction in the overall expenses paid through an employer-based plan. Examples of incentives to employees enjoying excellent health as identified from key biometric measures such as blood pressure and body weight include reductions in health insurance premiums or receipt of rewards and premium discounts for employees who have never smoked. Each of these efforts is designed to promote financial rewards to those who will likely not expose the organization to high health-care expenses in the future. From the KFF/HRET Survey, 83 percent of employer-based plans offer some form of incentive to promote wellness and disease prevention, with some firms having on-site programs that promote relaxation, stress reduction, and alternative medicine therapies that have the secondary benefit of enhancing workforce productivity.

  Still other employers reduce their share of premium exposure by designing benefit structures that address some of the fastest-growing and highest-expense components of twenty-first century health care. One such expense is in modifying health insurance plan designs for pharmaceutical expenses, where significant medication cost exposure has resulted from coverage of medications arising from research, development, and marketing of newer, high-cost drugs. An example of a high-expense medication is the recent discovery of Harvoni for treatment of chronic hepatitis C, an acquired infectious disease of the liver found in large enough numbers of baby boomers that recommendations have been publicized by the US Preventive Health Task Force to screen all persons born between 1946 and 1964.[169] According to recent reports, Harvoni costs $94,500 for a twelve-week course but is 90 percent effective in eradicating a disease that can result in liver

---

169 "Testing Recommendations for Hepatitis C Virus Infection," *Centers for Disease Control and Prevention: Viral Hepatitis,* accessed May 17, 2017, https://www.cdc.gov/hepatitis/hcv/guidelinesc.htm.

failure or liver cancer.[170] Some plans have limited its use for the sickest of patients with hepatitis C, while others have viewed the administration of Harvoni through the same cost-benefit analysis lens as cancer chemotherapy, where costs frequently approach $100,000 per year. Some employers have begun to design pharmaceutical benefit structures that require greater contributions from their workers in the form of higher premiums or higher deductibles, leading to greater out-of-pocket contributions from workers.

If employer-based insurance is to continue, innovative approaches from employers are needed for these plans to remain financially solvent. In addition to cost-shifting plan premiums toward employees, several other strategies have been incorporated into employer plan design and administration over the years, including:

- *Value-based purchasing.* Many employers have routinely negotiated with insurance companies or with provider networks regarding the value created by the health systems that are offered as part of the plan's design. From trends noted in the KFF/HRET Survey, 6–9 percent of employers have dropped a health system due to quality and performance issues, while another 5–8 percent of employers have created extremely narrow provider networks with significant penalties for employee utilization outside those networks. Finally, between 17 and 24 percent of all employer-sponsored plans have created a tiered network approach where employees may use hospitals and health systems that have been strategically placed based on the value created from the premium dollars invested. This steerage had risen to prominence when point of service (POS) plans were the approach taken by employers attempting to offer choice for their employees while still

---

170 A. Harding, "Pros and Cons of New Hepatitis C Drugs," updated April 7, 2017, accessed March 27, 2017, *everydayhealth.com.*

applying some financial constraints on workers.[171] Like HMO plans, employees select a primary-care provider, but in a twist that makes the POS plan similar to a PPO, employees may choose to receive services outside the selected network, paying higher copayments or coinsurance. In these plans, choice is also balanced against higher premiums for such flexibility. Some years ago, I had the opportunity to speak with a benefits representative from General Motors, who suggested that their company provided steerage toward high-value providers by publishing data related to processes and outcomes from care along with the costs encountered in these experiences. The employees, seeing the data, understood why certain providers were placed in a higher out-of-pocket expense category than others, and quite often GM found shifts in employee demand for some providers over others based on these data, thereby reducing costs while simultaneously promoting high-quality care providers.

• **_Promoting telehealth approaches._** Several experiments in telemedicine have been attempted over the past thirty years, beginning with an NIH-grant-funded effort to provide access to dermatology services to rural counties to enhance access to the diagnostic acumen of specialty-care practices. From such early efforts that I helped evaluate in the mid-1990s in Iowa, ambulatory telemedicine and telehealth solutions have continued to have an audience. Several examples of telemedicine services are now being used routinely, such as providing access to tertiary and quaternary care specialists from high-performing health systems such as the Mayo Clinic Care Network, thereby reducing the travel costs associated with a visit to south-central Minnesota.[172] Still other efforts have been promoted at job sites where primary-care telemedicine encounters have been provided in hope of reducing the time

---

171 "Point of Service (POS) Plans," HealthCare.gov, accessed May 17, 2017, https://www. healthcare.gov/glossary/point-of-service-plan-POS-plan/.

172 Mayo Clinic News Network, "Telemedicine & You: Mayo Clinic Expert Explains New Health Care Option, How State and National Policies Can Catch Up," January 29, 2015, accessed May 17, 2017, http://newsnetwork.mayoclinic.org/discussion/telemedicine-you-mayo-clinic-expert-explains-new-health-care-option-how-policy-can-catch-up/.

spent away from work to travel to and from a primary-care visit and reducing long wait times in remote physician offices. These telemedicine efforts have been contractually guaranteed either at discounted fee-for-service rates or for a monthly subscription rate, both with the purpose of reducing the total cost of care while also promoting access to highly effective and efficient health-care services. In general, both providers and consumers of care have held these visits in high regard, as they address the key driver of convenience for both groups.[173,174]

- *Modifying pharmaceutical coverage design.* As mentioned above, pharmaceutical costs are some of the most rapidly growing expenses in the spectrum of health-care services. To keep pharma costs in check, companies have adopted additional strategies to control costs aside from simple cost shifting to their employees. Some companies have commissioned special "carve outs" where an independent company assumes risk for the medication costs to treat certain expensive clinical conditions such as cancer care. Having specialized expertise, these carve-out companies manage drug expenses by promoting the use of evidence-based approaches that are typically accompanied by a gainsharing arrangement with health-care providers. By incorporating best practices into every encounter for treatment of cancer, for example, the resultant savings can be shared between the company and the provider if clinical outcomes are demonstrated to be superior.

Another check on costly medication use is defining a step-care approach to access high-cost medications. Instead of a provider being allowed to initiate care with a very expensive medication, some companies have been successful in having providers prescribe less costly but still appropriate medications as initial therapy. If those choices prove to be ineffective, then the next "step" in the treatment algorithm

173 J.L.Davis,"TelemedicineOffersPatientSatisfaction,"WebMD,May28,2002,accessedMay17, 2017, http://www.webmd.com/women/news/20020528/telemedicine-offers-patient-satisfaction.

174 K. Collins, P. Nicolson, and I. Bowns, "Patient Satisfaction in Telemedicine" (abstract), *Health Informatics Journal*, June 1, 2000, accessed May 17, 2017, http://journals.sagepub.com/doi/abs/10.1177/146045820000600205.

can be prescribed so that the greatest value can be obtained from the care experience, balancing the clinical outcome against a lower medication cost. Still other health plans promote purchasing efficiencies by encouraging employees to use mail-order pharmacies to purchase three months of a medication prescription to yield reductions in the monthly cost of medications when purchased in bulk.[175] This strategy is highly effective for medications purchased to treat stable chronic conditions, but it does not work as well when frequent changes are needed to a medication regimen. Similar to this, but not currently advocated by employer-based plans, is the ability to purchase medications from Canada and the European Union, where medication costs are much lower for identical drugs. Long a matter of debate between pharmaceutical companies and insurance providers, purchasing medications at a steep discount from sources outside the United States has been a successful strategy used by a number of Americans vacationing in foreign lands, although the practice has been discouraged by pharmaceutical manufacturers due to potential safety concerns from a company's inability to validate the authenticity of a particular medication purchased from a distributor not tied directly to the manufacturer.

One final approach used to reduce pharmaceutical costs where contracting terms are used as a key driver is in the creation of a multitier approach to medication prescribing, where some drugs are covered by the plan with a minimum deductible, while others have higher coinsurance costs to the individual patient. Examples of medications found in the lower tier of costs are generic drugs, where pricing is typically quite low and financial incentives are offered by the health plan, such as zero copayment or very low copayment or coinsurance. Higher-priced brand-name drugs occupy a higher tier on a medication formulary and have much higher out-of-pocket contributions

175 K. M. Robinson, "Online and Mail-Order Medicine: How to Buy Safely," WebMD, accessed May 4, 2017, http://www.webmd.com/healthy-aging/features/beyond-the-pharmacy-online-and-mail-order-prescription-drugs#1.

from patients, leaving the health-care consumer in a position to negotiate with a provider to secure the highest value for the out-of-pocket
dollars invested in medications.

- **_Embracing retail health care._** With the ascent of retail health-care
  providers found in big-box department stores or retail pharmacies,
  employers are now exploring relationships with lower-cost providers
  for evaluation and treatment of common medical conditions. Initially
  called "retail health providers" because they did not accept insurance
  coverage and relied on credit-card transactions for payment, their relationships with health plans have strengthened as they have shifted
  from "competitor" to "collaborator" in an effort to promote these
  lower-cost sites of service. The use of retail providers to administer
  annual immunizations such as influenza and pneumonia vaccination
  was an initial foray into the high-value nature of retail services, and in
  many areas of the country, retail services are now becoming fully integrated with traditional health-care providers so that each site can provide services appropriate for licensure while keeping patient records
  connected using an electronic health record interface.

One further impact on employer-provided insurance is being felt by employers
that provide extremely rich health-care benefit designs, colloquially referred to
as "Cadillac" plans. The Affordable Care Act looked to impart a special tax
on such plans to level the playing field for ERISA plans, which had unique
ability to offer atypical benefits that not only could attract high-performing
employees but would be tax deductible as well, creating a "double win" for certain employers with the means to offer such rich benefit designs.[176] From the
KFF/HRET Employer Survey, only 53 percent of employers have performed
the analysis and test of whether their plan offerings would be rich enough
to be called a "Cadillac plan," and 19 percent of those who had performed

---

176 J. Gold, "'Cadillac' Insurance Plans Explained," *Kaiser Health News*, January 15, 2010, accessed May 9, 2017, http://khn.org/news/cadillac-health-explainer-npr/.

the analysis found that they would be subjected to an additional tax.[177] In response, such qualifying employers have contemplated lowering the richness of benefit design to embrace greater employee cost sharing or considered shifting to high-deductible health plans with health savings accounts. Much like what occurred in the 1990s with pension plan benefits and the shift from defined benefit to defined contribution plans, there is an anticipated shift in employer health plan designs that serves as a defensive financial strategy to balance the company's desire to provide health-care coverage for employees against the negative impact on financial margins that will arise from continuing rich benefit packages. Health-care benefits, as important as they are to most employees, are beginning to be considered as a portion of a full spectrum of employee benefits so that the greatest value can be attained by the greatest number of workers at a cost that allows a firm to remain in business. The impact on health-care consumers and their relationship with health-care providers has been significant, with both parties beginning to view the consumption of health-care services much as they would the purchase of any other commodity such as salt, milk, and gasoline. ·

177 *Kaiser/HRET Survey of Employer-Sponsored Health Benefits, 1999–2015*, accessed March 27, 2017.

Key Points to Master From Chapter 9

- Although employer-sponsored health insurance began in 1789, but it was not until the 1920's that such plans became popular in the United States, becoming highly valued during a time when the economy was booming and insurance plans served to competitively advantage a company against loss of skilled employees.
- COBRA (the Consolidated Omnibus Budget Reconciliation Act) was passed in 1965 to offer employees a degree of financial security if they had suffered through a period of coverage loss arising from job loss tied to relocation, termination, or from a global reduction in workforce.
- The Employee Retirement Income Security Act (ERISA) of 1974 provided regulations that defined the documentation required by employers choosing to direct the administration of health benefits provided in their own work site.
- Key trends in employer health insurance provision from data collected by the Kaiser Family Foundation and the Health Research & Educational Trust include:
  o Trends in sources of health insurance coverage
  o Trends in health benefit design and administration
  o Trends in premium cost sharing
  o Special issues that impact health insurance such as wellness and prevention programs and coverage of expensive medications.
- Innovative approaches to maintain employer-sponsored health plan solvency:
  o Value based purchasing to reward the value of health care
  o Promotion of telehealth to reduce costs of care and worker absenteeism
  o Modifying benefit design for high cost pharmaceutical agents such as biologicals and injectable medications.
  o Embracing retail health care to lower the unit cost of preventive care and evaluation and treatment of minor conditions.

Ten

THE ROLES OF THE FEDERAL GOVERNMENT

On February 28, 2017, President Donald J. Trump announced at a meeting of the nation's governors at the White House that "we have come up with a solution that's really, really I think very good." He went on to say, "Now I have to tell you, it's an unbelievably complex subject. Nobody knew that health care could be so complicated."[178] That same day, Speaker of the House Representative Paul Ryan stated that the Republican majority was on a "rescue mission" to help protect Americans from the folly that had been put in place in 2010 as the Patient Protection and Affordable Care Act (ACA), affectionately known as "Obamacare."[179] When the Republican authors failed to garner enough votes to bring the bill in front of the full House, Ryan was instructed by Trump to pull the bill from consideration. Falling to an old Washington saying, "First you get the votes, then you take the vote,"[180] the Republican majority found itself trapped between two opposing forces within their party.

---

178 K. Liptak, *CNN Politics*, February 28, 2017, accessed March 28, 2017, http://www.cnn.com/2017/02/27/politics/trump-health-care-complicated/index.html.

179 J. Crowe, "Paul Ryan: 'We're on a Rescue Mission' for Obamacare," *Newsmax*, February 28, 2017, accessed May 17, 2017, http://www.newsmax.com/politics/paul-ryan-rescue-mission-obamacare/2017/02/28/id/776016/.

180 A. Prokop, *Vox Topics*, Trending, March 24, 2017, accessed March 28, 2017, http://www.vox.com/2017/3/24/15014202/house-ahca-vote-canceled-trump.

On the extreme right were representatives of the conservative Freedom Caucus, who criticized the bill's authors for keeping too many vestiges of Obamacare that had provided rich benefits for people who had recently been able to access health-care coverage through expanded Medicaid funding or through federal subsidies, allowing them to purchase a plan on the health insurance exchanges.[181] On the more moderate front, some Republicans, gathering under the name of the Tuesday Group, feared that many of their constituents would lose coverage under the proposal, perhaps costing them seats in the 2018 midterm elections.[182]

The case above illustrates the complexity of the federal government's operations, where some wonder how anything ever gets accomplished given the many and varied interests being represented in our beautiful republican form of government with its three equal branches. Complicating this intricate process, many rules of order can flip dramatically based on an election that brings sweeping change to a majority/minority balance in Congress nearly overnight. When the framers of the Constitution brought forth the idea of a representative democracy that markedly differed from the previous ruling British monarchy, the belief was that while it might be messy and require debate and much hand-wringing to get laws passed, its strength was the very fact that it required consensus following respectful debate to bring resolution to political and social issues. It was the hope of our founders that the democratic experiment that was the United States of America should reinforce issue resolution when elected representatives' interests transcend cronyism and personal privilege.

The World Health Organization (WHO) defines health policy as "the decisions, plans, and actions that are undertaken to achieve specific healthcare goals within a society."[183] The WHO continues, "An explicit health policy can

---

181 D. Weigel, "Freedom Caucus Backs ACA 'Repeal and Replace' That Counts on Private Health Care," *Washington Post*, February 15, 2017.

182 C. A. Williams, M. W. Truax, K. Griffith, and A. M. Redman, "House GOP Clings to ACA Repeal Dream Despite Bill Collapse," *Benefit News*, March 28, 2017, accessed May 17, 2017, https://www.benefitnews.com/articles/house-gop-clings-to-aca-repeal-dream-despite-bill-collapse.

183 World Health Organization, "Health Policy," accessed March 28, 2017, http://www.who.int/topics/health_policy/en/.

achieve several things: it defines a vision for the future which in turn helps to establish targets and points of reference for the short and medium term. It outlines priorities and the expected roles of different groups; and it builds consensus and informs people." Health policy is quite expansive and inclusive, encompassing the delivery and financing of health care, the quality and safety of care delivered, and issues associated with access to care and health equity. It is no wonder, then, that health-care legislation has been historically very difficult to successfully implement, since so many of the people involved with legislating are also influenced by sectors representing the many different special-interest views of the topics covered under the banner of health policy. Just like the example of a group of blind men attempting to guess the identity of an animal as an elephant when each has grasped only one small piece of the beast, comprehensive health-care financing solutions are quite difficult to debate and resolve. Typically, when one aspect of health-care financing or access is modified, several other equally important unanticipated consequences can arise.

Health policy debate and the resultant rules, regulations, and laws that arise from such debate can generate changes to a health-care delivery system that are well beyond the preferences of providers and consumers. For health-care providers, evidence-based studies are the measuring stick used to define the value of a new program, with outcomes able to be directly measured as part of a "cause and effect" deployment of an intervention under study. For health-care consumers, some deference to expertise can be seen as providers are given great latitude to demonstrate what works best, with the consumer focus largely based on whether a health-care experience was successful in generating great value for the out-of-pocket costs. For federal and state officials, however, the health-care system construction and payment for services can be much less easily measured and much more complex than initially considered, since social, financial, and political forces all come together to create an ideology that frames political discourse. Further complicating the health-care policy debate is the fact that the philosophical construct of adding or removing programs involves the individual rights of their constituents, ethical decision-making, and the specter of government authority and reach. Since Congress represents groups of constituents who have had unique experiences that frame their personal views about health care, agreement on policies affecting health-care delivery are among some of the most complex on Capitol Hill. Complicating this ideological debate further, the health-care industrial complex now represents one-fifth of the gross domestic product of the United States, and any change to such a massive industry is certainly felt as shuddering ramifications in several other supporting sectors.[184,185]

This book is not intended to be a treatise on health policy, nor is it designed to serve as a political-science textbook. I do hope to frame the health-care debate that has occurred for decades to cast some light on many roles that the federal government plays in helping define and modify the relationship between health-care provider and health-care consumer. The hope is that if providers and consumers can agree on how health-care delivery systems should provide care with a focus on effectiveness, efficiency, patient-centeredness, and equity for all, they may be able to influence the national health-care debate as a united front. Rather than sitting passively on the sidelines as the government defines the evolving health-care relationship, it is the desire of many that providers and consumers will lead these debates. Simply stated, no other individuals have more to gain from a high-value health-care delivery system than health-care consumers and providers, and no individuals have more to lose from a system that has been poorly designed by politicians acting in isolation from those who use health-care systems.

On November 19, 1945, only seven months into his presidency, President Harry S. Truman introduced the idea that all Americans should have access to excellent health-care services.[186] Truman's proposal called for federal funding to support the salaries of physicians, nurses, dentists, and other health professionals to encourage their relocation to rural and poor counties to assist

184 V. R. Fuchs, "The Gross Domestic Product and Health Care Spending," *New England Journal of Medicine* 369, no. 3 (2013): 107–109.

185 National Health Expenditure Accounts (NHEA), Centers for Medicare and Medicaid Services, accessed May 17, 2017, https://www.cms.gov/Research-Statistics-Data-and-Systems/Statistics-Trends-and-Reports/NationalHealthExpendData/NationalHealthAccountsHistorical.html.

186 Harry S. Truman Library & Museum, University of Missouri, *This Day in Truman History*, accessed March 28, 2017, https://www.trumanlibrary.org/anniversaries/healthprogram.htm.

in providing better access to care for all, regardless of geography or personal economy. Seeing that hospitals were similarly absent from rural and economically challenged parts of the country, Truman called for federal funding to assist in construction projects for new, higher-quality hospitals that would operate according to a set of standards implemented by a National Health Board made up of physicians and public officials. In addition to defining the standards of operation, the board would measure compliance to those standards and would direct funding for medical research. The final piece of Truman's proposal was the most controversial, calling for a national health insurance plan that was designed to cover all Americans, but it did not force anyone into participating in such a plan. Participants would be required to pay a monthly fee into the national health-care account, and all medical services would be paid to participating physicians from that account. Additional federal funding would be provided to cover any shortfall and to provide cash payments to plan participants who may have missed work or suffered from economic hardship. In response to such a radical proposal, the American Medical Association (AMA) lashed out against the plan, claiming that it was "socialized medicine" and should be viewed as a step toward communism.[187] Given the political sensitivities of Americans following World War II and the early calls for congressional hearings on treason and subversives that were emanating from Senator Joe McCarthy's office, it was no wonder that the proposal met an untimely death, particularly when Truman's staff were called "followers of the Moscow party line" in AMA publications.[188]

Since Truman's initial proposal calling for national health insurance with coverage for all Americans, there have been three additional failures over the past sixty years that predated the Affordable Care Act's passage in 2010. Former Senator Tom Daschle, writing in a 2008 publication, stated that political efforts at implementing a health policy solution that addressed the needs

187 L. Cushing, "A History of Total Health: Kaiser Permanente as a National Model for Care," July 22, 2015, accessed May 16, 2017, http://kaiserpermanentehistory.org/tag/american-medical-association/.

188 K. Doherty and J. A. Jenkins, "Examining a Failed Moment: National Health Care, the AMA, and the U.S. Congress, 1948–50," January 7, 2009, accessed May 9, 2017, http://faculty.virginia.edu/jajenkins/health_care.pdf.

of all Americans have failed on multiple occasions because of a combination of health-care delivery system complexity, limitations of the political system itself, and the power of special-interest groups that have a direct stake in the outcome of any political solution.[189] Daschle called out doctors, hospitals, insurers, drug companies, researchers, and even patient advocates for being complicit in the country's inability to provide health-care access to millions of people who are mired in debt due to their inability to pay medical bills in the absence of health insurance.

Since the publication of Daschle's book, a Democrat-led assault on health-care coverage resulted in the Patient Protection and Accountable Care Act, which went to President Barrack Obama for signature in early 2010. Both sides of the aisle agree that several aspects of "Obamacare" remain in need of fine-tuning, but the morass of political ideology that is the federal government prevents discussion of how the act might be improved, rather promoting a focus on how to repeal all of the ACA provisions to start anew. As calls came from the conservative right for a full repeal of the legislation without any replacement, Democrats feared what the full repeal of the plan might mean to millions of Americans who had just recently become insured. More moderate Republicans called for a "repeal and replace" or a "repair and replace" approach to the nation's first successful effort at universal coverage, recognizing that many people who elected them to serve would likely be affected adversely in the wake of the elimination of some of the coverage provisions that would result in loss of coverage for as many as twenty-four million Americans.[190]

So, what are the intrinsic limitations of our political reality that interrupt the path forward in debating how best to approach health-care coverage solutions in the United States?

- *Ideology and special interests.* Campaigns for election and reelection have become near-continuous events, and the appearance of yard

---

189 T. Daschle, *Critical: What We Can Do about the Health-Care Crisis* (Thomas Dunne Books, 2008).

190 Congressional Budget Office, *American Health Care Act*, March 13, 2017, accessed May 6, 2017, https://www.cbo.gov/publication/52486.

signs, political stump speeches, and requests for contributions have yielded a political system where the most important job of a representative is to ensure his or her reelection. Before tightened regulations on the "pork barrel constituency" in Congress, it was not unusual for members to trade earmarks for votes,[191] and powerful influence was created through a series of horse trades between congressional representatives. These negotiations produced additions to proposed bills that could demonstrate the effectiveness of a congressperson back home in his or her district if a new bridge were funded for construction, and these additional perks were frequently named for popular folk heroes from the district. In today's political climate, the key to reelection is the "power of the purse," and candidates frequently build up huge war chests to create political infrastructures that make challenges to incumbents quite costly and less likely to be successful.

The tides clearly changed in 2010 when the United States Supreme Court ruled that corporations and unions could pay for political ads if they were made independent of formal campaign structures, thereby reversing the McCain-Feingold law of 2002, which had been a bipartisan effort to limit the impact of corporate influence on elections.[192] Although federal campaign finance reform dates back to the Civil War, the Supreme Court ruling on a narrow vote allowed greater influence by representatives of powerful lobbying groups, and health-care legislation has seen its share of political influence in the few short years since corporate donations began to influence elections.

Two examples help illustrate the ways in which special-interest financing has helped create political tides regarding health-care legislation. The first is the recognition that the greater the potential loss of corporate and individual revenues from changes to legislation, the greater the impetus to provide funding that will influence the

---

191 R. Longley, "What Is Earmark Spending in the US Congress," *ThoughtCo.*, January 5, 2016, accessed May 9, 2017, https://www.thoughtco.com/what-is-earmark-spending-in-congress-3322285.
192 Adam Liptak, "Justices, 5–4, Reject Corporate Spending Limit," *New York Times*, January 21, 2010, accessed March 28, 2017.

outcome of a proposed bill. Daschle cites the impact of contributions from the pharmaceutical industry that influenced health-care legislation, stating that "between 1998 and 2006, pharmaceutical companies and other manufacturers of health-care products spent over a billion dollars on lobbying, more than anybody else and twice as much as the oil and gas industries. Insurance companies, including health insurers, ranked second."[193] A second example occurred in the response to efforts to pass the American Health Care Act, which was due to be voted on by the full House of Representatives in March 2017. According to reports published by the New York *Daily News* on March 23, 2017, Charles and David Koch announced through their advocacy networks that they would create a new fund for GOP representatives who voted against the White House-backed legislation.[194] Many other influences exist on Capitol Hill, and the lobbyists representing numerous protected classes of people who have a vested interest in preserving the status quo are quite plentiful. Powerful by virtue of their large numbers of members, groups such as AARP, which represents over thirty-eight million people over the age of fifty, can exert tremendous influence as highly engaged voters speak together with a single and powerful voice about issues such as resisting any change to existing Medicare provisions.[195]

- *Gerrymandering and preservation of status.* In a 2016 State of the Union address, President Obama called for an end to gerrymandering, the process of redrawing district lines in a way that may favor one group selectively over another.[196] He stated, "We have to end the practice of drawing our congressional districts so that politicians can

193 Daschle, *Critical: What We Can Do about the Health-Care Crisis.*

194 C. Sommerfeldt, "Koch Brothers Reportedly Pledge Millions to Republicans Opposing Trump-Backed Health Care Bill," *New York Daily News*, March 23, 2017, accessed March 28, 2017.

195 AARP, "Make a Difference," accessed May 17, 2017, http://www.aarp.org/about-aarp/.

196 J. Fabian, "Obama: Gerrymandering Stokes Gridlock in Congress," *The Hill*, August 10, 2015.

pick their voters, rather than the other way around."[197] When an election district is drawn with unusual geographic boundaries to preserve that district's hold on a congressional seat, and if term limits are not in place, it is not unusual to see preservation of the status quo, and there is little chance of rebalancing the political ideologies that drive the current state forward. As long as politicians understand the mathematical equation needed to win reelection, the voices of the many may be drowned out by the voices of the few who have a vested interest in maintaining the political climate of their district. Resistance to change is not just a barrier to improvements needed in health-care quality and safety, but it is a universal human tendency that creates political scenarios leading to little real change, particularly in congressional district ideology.

- *Health care is "too big to fail."* As health-care delivery systems and health insurance companies move through inevitable consolidation, these institutions become of such a grand scale that they are viewed as being too big to fail for fear of the impact of their failure on the global United States economy. A moral hazard is created when an industry takes advantages of its economic influence to create an environment where companies can leverage profits from the preferred position they occupy in legislative circles. Seen clearly in 2007–2008 when the banking industry was engaged in high-risk, high-reward behaviors, when the economic crash inevitably occurred, some banking institutions were viewed as being "too big to fail" and the impact too disastrous without some financial assistance provided by the federal government. Similarly, when the health-care industrial complex grows at the rate that it has over the past half century, it now rivals all other sectors for a protected status given the consequences that might arise should significant changes be proposed to provide cost controls on the systems of production. The weight of such an impact sits heavily on politicians' shoulders, leading to a great deal of caution when they

---

197 C. Ingraham, "This Is Actually What America Would Look Like Without Gerrymandering," *Washington Post*, January 13, 2016, accessed March 28, 2017.

consider potential recommendations for change to a system where expenses are rising at rapid rates and outcomes are not keeping pace with federal government's expenditures. This imbalance results in a continued drag on the nation's economy and its reputation as the world's most technologically advanced and innovative country.

- *"Perfect is the enemy of good."* This saying is just as true today as it was when it was popularized by Voltaire in 1770. A focus on making health-care legislation perfect at every turn can produce stalemates and quagmires that keep any changes from occurring, producing legislative inertia. Many politicians cite the impact they feel from stories relayed to them in their home districts that describe the many ways that having little or no insurance coverage affects the average American. These adverse impacts are felt personally by those individuals who are harmed when they do not have access to preventive health care or when they experience delays in diagnosis of serious conditions. Trying to create perfect solutions to existing problems, the "perfect" legislation is frequently attacked when lack of congruence in political platform is achieved during debate with legislators from other locations. When the United States was a much smaller and less complex society, these differences could be easily ironed out through respectful debate, but today's nuanced communities have produced a political climate where debate is vociferous, disjointed, and less productive.

Constituents understand the real issues being experienced by their friends and neighbors, as shown by polling evidence that has demonstrated growing acceptance and approval of the Affordable Care Act.[198] From its initial passage, the ACA did not enjoy great favorability, with more than 50 percent of Americans viewing the health-care bill poorly, and as health-care premiums began to rise in 2014, there was a significant negative perception of the ACA

---

198 "Public Approval of Health Care Law," Real Clear Politics, March 14, 2017, accessed March 28, 2017, http://www.realclearpolitics.com/epolls/other/obama_and_democrats_health_care_plan-1130.html.

with a 13.2 percent spread between those opposing the bill and those supporting it.[199] This changed markedly when the "repeal and replace" legislation in the House of Representatives was being publicly discussed, and at the time when the proposal was being readied for vote, the average of all polls demonstrated that more Americans supported the existing legislation than when it was originally signed in 2010.[200]

Many solutions to the health-care spending crisis have been offered, largely along ideological lines, with little hope of any of them creating sustainable solutions. The idea of securing the political will while maintaining the ability to engage in debate is as important today as it was when our framers hammered out the most magnificent and complex document that described the very origins of this country. Not perfect in its construction, the Constitution came forth through the airing of multiple viewpoints and vigorously debated differences of opinion. The essential elements that helped bring this great document to life included a focus on servant leadership, reliance on a sense of political morality that reflects the wishes of the country, and a focus on what will help the majority of the country without getting mired down in an effort to create a "perfect" legislative masterpiece. Therein lies the test for our political representatives: can these elected representatives of the people find a way for respectful bipartisan debate to exist with comity lighting the path toward a set of solutions that can be then be amended as needed in the future?

---

199 S. Shepard, "Poll: Support for Obamacare Is Rising," *Politico*, February 22, 2017.

200 Kaiser Family Foundation, "Kaiser Health Tracking Poll: The Public's Views on the ACA," accessed May 17, 2017, http://kff.org/interactive/kaiser-health-tracking-poll-the-publics-views-on-the-aca/#?response=Favorable--Unfavorable&aRange=twoYear.

Key Points to Master From Chapter 10

- In 1945, President Harry S. Truman called for federal funding to support the salaries of physicians, nurses, dentists, and other health professionals to encourage their relocation to rural and poor counties to assist in providing better access to care for all. The plan called for assistance with construction of new, higher-quality hospitals operating according to a set of standards implemented by a National Health Board made up of physicians and public officials. The final piece of Truman's proposal was the most controversial, calling for development of a national health insurance plan.
- The debate about federal health insurance has come to the fore in nearly all administrations, ranging from Medicare during the Johnson years to a Nixon proposal for comprehensive health care coverage, to Clinton's Health Security Plan, Obama's Affordable Care Act, and Trump's American Health Care Act.
- Three distinct approaches were debated following the 2016 election:
  o Modify the ACA through funding that would lower insurance premiums
  o Repeal and replace the ACA with a more flexible, market-based approach
  o Repeal the ACA and start anew the task of creating a federal plan
- Key limitations found in the political debate concerning health insurance:
  o Divisive ideologies exist that have significant ties to health care financing proposals provided by special interest advocacy efforts.
  o Gerrymandering preserves the *status quo* and entrenches the divisions
  o Health care, like banking, has become "too big to fail"
  o "Perfect is the enemy of good enough"
- The Affordable Care Act has grown in acceptance and favorability as working-class Americans begin to understand the potential losses in coverage that come with passage of the American Health Care Act.

Eleven

EVOLUTION OF THE SOCIAL COMPACT FOR CARE

D r. Bruno Masters, one of my earliest mentors, served as the program director for my residency program in family medicine. On the first day of orientation, he came to address the bright and shiny faces that covered up our intense feelings of incompetence mixed with incredibly low levels of confidence that we all shared in preparing to start the long journey toward becoming a "real doctor." Dr. Masters helped us feel much more at home when he informed us, in his best Southern drawl acquired from years of practice in North Carolina, that his primary job was to "help us all to grow up enough to earn the responsibility of caring for another human being." He relayed that we had been psychologically stunted by years of pursuing useless information arising from endless memorization of facts about organic chemistry, physics, and calculus, and that these long hours of late-night study had rendered us frozen at the emotional age of a young teenager. His most important job was to help us become more human in our professional pursuits, capable of earning the special bond with patients who would grow to rely on us as much for our comforting reassurances as for our medical diagnoses.

Believing we were to undergo a complete physical examination as part of our residency orientation, we were each led to an exam room and instructed that a senior resident would be with us shortly to complete the requisite procedure. Concealed was a well-planned experience that Dr. Masters had created for us, giving us firsthand knowledge about what it felt like to be a patient. This memorable moment served as an example of a "cold" medical-care experience, and he was assisted by his faculty, resident physicians, and nursing staff, who each reinforced key components of a disastrous patient office encounter. The nursing staff gave us little explanation of what was to come next, telling us only to take off all our clothes and to be seated on a cold metal exam table that had been imported solely for this experience. Every few minutes, the exam room door cracked open without warning, and no apology was offered for the undesired interruption, nor was any explanation given for what was to happen next. Sitting on the cold chromed surface for fifteen minutes left me shivering. Finally, the examining resident came into the room and immediately placed a refrigerator-chilled stethoscope on my chest, telling me to breathe in and out as he harrumphed his way through the examination. He left silently after a cursory exam, answering no questions and leaving me with no instructions about what to do next or what findings he would record in my newly minted medical record. Ten more minutes passed before a faculty member came into the room and told me to get dressed and go to the conference room for a debriefing. Walking dejectedly into the conference room, cursing myself for the terrible mistake I had made by selecting the Iowa Lutheran residency program over what had been a very appropriate second choice, I was greeted by a group of smiling residents and faculty members who were offering free coffee and breakfast sandwiches. Only then were we let in on the lesson that had been provided to us, one that plainly demonstrated a powerful reminder about the importance of patient dignity, respect, and communication. Thus began the journey toward "actual doctoring," as Dr. Masters called it—the realization that despite all the science and technical knowledge we needed to acquire, we had entered into a unique profession that was most importantly tied to a special bond created between two individuals, one human providing health-care services and another human in search of a compassionate care experience.

On June 13, 2016, the American Medical Association updated its *Code of Medical Ethics*, the first update to the document in more than fifty years.[201] Initially created in 1847, the AMA's position paper became the first of its kind for any professional group, and updates that have been introduced over the years have addressed a profession that continues to become more complex and diversified in its practices and its member representatives. The resulting *Code of Medical Ethics* begins with a section entitled "Patient-Physician Relationships," which describes the practice of medicine as the embodiment of a clinical encounter that is fundamentally a moral activity.[202] It defines the experience as a duty focusing on provision of care for a patient and how a caregiver should relieve suffering based on a trust-based relationship where a physician places a patient's welfare above the physician's own self-interests or obligations to others. In a separate section on communication and decision-making, physicians are reminded that patients have "the right to receive information and ask questions about recommended treatments so they can make well-considered decisions about care." Physicians are counseled to uphold the standards of the profession, and if laws or regulations are proposed that are contrary to the best interest of patients, physicians are to seek changes in those requirements to keep patients' interests at the forefront of each care experience. The final two ethical principles from the 2016 revision call for physicians to consider their commitment to patient care paramount and to support access to medical care for all people, regardless of standing in the community.

Previously, a physician charter had been created in work performed by the Medical Professionalism Project,[203] a coalition of physicians representing the American Board of Internal Medicine, the American College of Physicians,

---

201 S. Brotherton, A. Kao, and B. J. Crigger, "Professing the Values of Medicine: The Modernized AMA Code of Medical Ethics," *Journal of the American Medical Association* 316, no. 10 (2016): 1041–1042.

202 American Medical Association, *Code of Medical Ethics*, accessed April 3, 2017, http://www.ama-assn.org.

203 "Medical Professionalism in the New Millennium: A Physician Charter," *Annals of Internal Medicine* 136, no. 3 (2002): 243–246.

and the European Federation of Internal Medicine. Published in 2002, the charter served to remind physicians that health-care organizational changes sometimes threaten the value of professionalism and that certain conditions in medical practice were evolving that could tempt physicians to abandon their commitment to the primacy of patient welfare. Three main principles were professed in the Medical Professionalism Project document:

- **Primacy of patient welfare.** Based on trust and altruism, this principle was placed first because of the importance of maintaining a several-hundred-year history of caregivers upholding a commitment to the best interests of a person seeking assistance, and because this personal and professional calling was to remain at the center of medical-care experiences without erosion from market forces, societal pressures, or administrative conflicts. Founded in the Hippocratic Oath[204] and reinforced to all caregivers as a pristine and unshakeable commitment to the phrase "patients first," the primacy of patient welfare has guided the health-care profession through some of the most complicated economic, political, and societal challenges faced throughout the history of the profession.
- **Patient autonomy.** Keeping with the principle of patient welfare primacy, autonomy implies that no decision should be made without incorporating the input of the person receiving care. It promotes practitioner honesty and a commitment to engaging patients in their own care decisions through an empowered relationship that incorporates the best thinking of both the person providing care and the person receiving care. It assumes information flow through effective communication methods and places patient decision-making paramount if the decisions being made are ethical and focused on appropriate health-care service delivery.
- **Social justice.** This principle calls for health-care providers to serve as advocates for persons in need, regardless of race, gender, socioeconomic

---

204 "The Hippocratic Oath, Modern Version," Johns Hopkins Sheridan Libraries & University Museums, accessed May 25, 2017, http://guides.library.jhu.edu/c.php?g=202502&p=1335759.

status, ethnicity, religion, or any other social category. It calls for a fair distribution of health-care resources and reinforces the Institute of Medicine's call for high-quality and high-value care by assuring equitability. As a former health system CEO once told me, "There can be no quality without equality."[205]

In outlining the three principles, the working group called for all physicians to restate their commitment to the communities in which they worked and lived, independent of the political and financial challenges that were being felt as part of health-care organizational reformation efforts arising at the turn of the millennium. The document counseled health-care providers to remain focused first on providing high-quality care. Although organizational interests might be in conflict with the more holistic principles of caring for the people of the community, physicians were charged with keeping their promise to care for and about anyone who is in need. With the recognition that corporate medical practice might blur the lines traditionally separating health-care organizations from private physician practices, the working group wanted to remind physicians that although health system culture, policies, and behaviors need to be embraced, there is a fine line between blindly following those tenets and losing sight of the sacrosanct provider-patient bond.

Helping bring all remaining parties to the cultural table, the Foundation for Medical Excellence provided guidance under the Organizational Professionalism Charter Project, outlined in March 2017, which called for sound policies to govern the evolution of health-care organizations.[206] The group that authored the recommendations hoped that it could be used by hospital and health system boards of trustees, policy makers, care providers, and community members as an aspirational guide to maintain focus on the core principle of promoting health by members of the healing professions. Four key areas cited to promote health included the development of patient

---

205 Quote attributed to Ram Raju, MD, former CEO of NYC Health & Hospitals, New York City, New York.
206 D. J. Mason, "Professionalism in Health Care Organizations," *Journal of the American Medical Association* 317, no. 12 (2017): 1203–1204.

partnerships, promotion of a culture of trust and empowerment, addressing social determinants of health through community partnership and collaboration, and attempting to focus on cost-effective health-care delivery without conflict of interest. The first of the four key focus areas reinforced the elements contained in the 2002 Physician Charter espoused by the American Board of Internal Medicine and was fully consistent with the AMA's modernized *Code of Ethics*. It called for shared decision-making following the transparent exchange of information between providers of care and consumers of care, confirming the values that define "what matters to patients" rather than simply asking them "what's the matter."

Discussions regarding organizational culture highlight the importance of mutual respect between health-care organizations and health-care workers that promotes diversity, teamwork, and a more globally healthy workforce. By addressing issues of health for the entire community, organizations are challenged to consider the social determinants of health for a community, such as housing, poverty, food insecurity, and violence. Supporting these tenets means building broad health collaboratives that are designed to promote a culture of health for an entire community, such as the recommendations being promoted by the Robert Wood Johnson Foundation.[207] Finally, to remind health-care organizations of the need to address their own operations to support more effective and efficient health-care delivery, the charter calls for health systems to conduct business transactions ethically, to promote patient privacy, to treat employees fairly, to address conflicts of interest appropriately, and to align organizational incentives with the values the health-care system expresses publicly.

Each of the three documents mentioned above centers on one unifying principle: maintaining the core elements of a centuries-old approach that is the social compact created between a provider of care services and a consumer of those services. At the very heart of the compact is an expression of caring for and about one another and maintaining a vigilant focus on the best interests of one another. The greatest challenge to this core principle is in the inevitable

---

207 "Building a Culture of Health," Robert Wood Johnson Foundation, accessed April 2, 2017, http://www.rwjf.org/en/how-we-work/building-a-culture-of-health.html.

distractions from its central theme that are found in life in the twenty-first century. When care providers, care consumers, policy makers, health insurance companies, health-care device manufacturers, and health-care administrators lose sight of the true mission of building greater health for a person and the community, the bond between provider and consumer can be strained or broken, and care outcomes can be compromised. To understand the overarching importance of the fragile provider-consumer compact and how it can be threatened, it is essential to review the research behind the benefits of such a relationship and the various ways in which this delicate relationship continues to evolve.

Does the provider-consumer relationship correlate in any way with improvement in clinical outcomes? Before efforts to quantify the elements that determine effectiveness of health-care outcomes, determinants of health were typically measured solely through the lens of the health-care provider. Consumers were not influential in proposing changes to care delivery systems, since they did not understand the health-care processes necessary to produce favorable clinical outcomes. But as per Adam Smith's "invisible hand" of consumer behaviors, a "perfect marketplace" would require information symmetry.[208] In other words, the buyer and seller of services must have the same information about those services for a reasonable transaction to exist. Since most people who participate as health-care consumers have little practical experience in diagnostics and therapeutics, they do not actively participate in their own strategies for care, and providers historically have embraced an approach of benevolent paternalism where decisions were made on behalf of patients, and patients simply deferred to the expertise of a caregiver.

As health-care financing began to change the nature of the relationship between care provider and care consumer, patients began asking for relevant and easily digestible information that would make them better health-care consumers. This had a significant impact on providers who were still operating in an environment where they were generally making decisions, and the actions to implement a treatment plan were carried out by the person who was

---

208 "Definition of 'Invisible Hand,'" *Economic Times*, accessed May 24, 2017, http://economictimes.indiatimes.com/definition/invisible-hand.

seeking a provider's advice. Intensifying this demand by patients to become more active participants in their own care was a call for greater autonomy by health-care consumers wishing to hold a more prominent seat at the decision-making table. Made easier by availability of medical information on the Internet and through patient support groups and discussion blogs, health-care consumers began asking providers for assistance in interpreting this expanding compendium of medical information. Rather than just deferring all health-care decisions to physicians, care consumers assumed that this information and their wishes would become incorporated into proposed treatment plans. This journey to become better-informed care consumers sometimes ended in strained relationships with their health-care providers. As some patients cited literature that was neither timely nor grounded in scientific theory, providers began to recoil from such requests, creating a stressful provider-consumer conversation.

One additional issue that arose from such efforts aimed at becoming better health-care consumers was the revelation that some providers did not always access the most current medical literature. Providers, caught off guard by requests to consider newer therapies, sometimes inappropriately minimized the value of studies being brought to their attention. The net effect of health-care consumers becoming more informed by mastering newly accessed medical information was a leveling of the playing field between doctor and patient, changing their historic relationship permanently.

Further complicating and changing the relationship between provider and consumer was the national movement to report publicly the outcomes of individual physicians, hospitals, and nursing homes on federal government sites such as Hospital Compare, which was managed by the Centers for Medicare and Medicaid Services.[209] With highly accessible reports that arose from surveys of patient experiences with care, procedure complication rates, readmission and mortality data by disease, and cost of care, the provider-consumer bond was further strained, since some physicians were strongly opposed to

---

209 "Hospital Compare," Centers for Medicare and Medicaid Services, accessed April 2, 2017, https://www.cms.gov/Medicare/Quality-Initiatives-Patient-Assessment-Instruments/Hospital QualityInits/HospitalCompare.html.

the publication of such data, viewing these public reports as biased and distasteful. Those same providers suggested that the patient care experience was being turned into a "retail transaction" that missed the nuances of differences in outcomes and experiences resulting from differences in the patient populations on which data was being reported. In addition to complaints from providers that the patients differed from one another in meaningful ways, providers expressed concerns about the methodology employed for surveying patients. Complaints were registered about how disease complications were being defined, since untoward outcomes arising from patient groups that had many comorbid medical conditions such as diabetes, heart disease, and geriatric frailty were not risk-adjusted and therefore were inaccurate. Finally, many providers felt that there was little or no correlation between the reported experiential data and the actual clinical outcomes for patients.

In a "Perspectives" column in 2013, Matthew Manary explored these questions to determine if provider complaints were well-founded or if these complaints were just a convenient excuse to abandon public reporting, especially the reporting of patient perceptions of care.[210] His group identified three main concerns that individuals had categorized related to patient care experiences that correlated imperfectly with clinical outcomes. The first concern was tied to the formulation of the survey itself with a feeling that patient experiences were being falsely measured, and what was being measured was actually a form of "generalized happiness" that could be influenced by any number of factors and not necessarily attributed to elements arising solely from the provider's contribution to the care experience. The second main complaint related to the observation that patients often fill out questionnaires without being able to directly correlate care processes with the questions they were being asked to complete. With literally hundreds and sometimes thousands of potential care decisions being made during an episode of care, some providers insisted that consumers were providing little feedback that correlated the care experience and the outcome from that experience. Finally, some providers pointed out that if a patient's specific desires were not met, such as the insistence on

210 M. P. Manary et al., "Perspective: The Patient Experience and Health Outcomes," *New England Journal of Medicine* 368 (2013): 201–203.

receiving a specific medication for which they had little medical grounds to request, then experience reporting would prove to be a poor correlate with clinical outcomes. As a case where care consumers are being asked for their opinions but not having those voices appreciated by some providers, a stalemate can be created, suggesting a need for further scientific study to establish the potential for correlation.

One area of study that does seem to have been well refined is related to satisfaction with the care experience and continuation of a treatment plan. Data from Jha and colleagues had earlier demonstrated good correlation between overall patient satisfaction with care and adherence to clinical guidelines for evidence-based care.[211] From data on evidence-based approaches, it was logical that use of evidence-based approaches was associated with improvement in clinical outcomes and reproducibly better care, and therefore higher degrees of patient satisfaction seemed likely to correlate to better outcomes. Other studies affirmed the relationship between patient satisfaction, hospital readmission rates,[212] and inpatient mortality.[213] In an audio interview regarding the use of patient reported data, Susan Edgman-Levitan suggests that patient-level data regarding health-care experiences are useful to help clinical teams uncover what care consumers value, what those consumers think would help manage their clinical conditions, and how those reflections could be used to define more effective overall health promotion strategies.[214] Although none of the studies mentioned above asked health-care consumers to delve deeply into the technical aspects of the health-care processes being deployed in their care plans, it does appear that the impressions of consumers track quite well with

211 A. K. Jha et al., "Patients' Perception of Hospital Care in the United States," *New England Journal of Medicine* 359 (2008): 1921–1931.

212 W. Boulding et al., "Relationship between Patient Satisfaction with Inpatient Care and Hospital Readmission within 30 Days," *American Journal of Managed Care* 17 (2011): 41–48.

213 S. W. Glickman et al., "Patient Satisfaction and Its Relationship with Clinical Quality and Inpatient Mortality in Acute Myocardial Infarction," *Circulation: Cardiovascular Quality Outcomes* 3 (2010): 188–195.

214 S. Egman-Levitan, audio interview in *New England Journal of Medicine*, accompanying vol. 368, pp. 201–203, accessed April 3, 2017.

their health outcomes, much to the chagrin of some providers who are not anxious to include an additional voice in therapeutic decision-making.

Additional influences on whether the consumer voice should occupy a seat at the new provider-consumer relationship table include commentary found in lay and specialty news outlets where "doctor celebrities" inform the public about clinical conditions, new medications, alternative and complementary therapies, and breakthroughs in research that are reported to yield new therapies for historically untreatable conditions. Direct-to-consumer advertising about medications has also created a demand for expensive brand-name pharmaceutical products that are suggested to be more effective than other remedies, with a careful caveat in each of these commercial advertisements that the patient should always discuss selection of medications with their personal physician. Newspapers and magazines also report on awards received by health-care institutions that can help differentiate some provider systems from their competitors based on an "objective" determination of quality and safety. Even employer-based health plans have stepped into the information age by providing web portals for employees to submit questions and receive answers to those queries before being authorized to visit a provider in person, thereby helping employees become better-informed health-care consumers.

From the health-care provider perspective, the relationship with the patient is shifting dramatically at a time when many other dissatisfiers aside from public reporting are also present. As the needs and demands from health-care consumers for greater amounts of information become commonplace, both providers and consumers want to become more tightly connected through information portals found in a patient's electronic health record. Providers became more comfortable with providing answers to patient questions using the asynchronous communication channels of an electronic patient portal that connects providers and consumers of care. Consumers began to ask questions about disease management strategies and health promotion and prevention activities, and they could do so without ever having to be seen by a provider. Some primary-care doctors reported seeing a growing number of office patients during the day and then continued their workday when they went home to answer an additional one to two hours of e-mail questions from their patients. A shift in reimbursement was being seen in most health systems that were employing physicians who had historically been independent practitioners, and payment models based on productivity were coming in vogue. More so than ever before, providers began seeing patient care visits as the main driver for their overall revenues, and many explored new care methods to see more patients in less time so that productivity could be maximized and financial incentives realized.

In a story originating from Kaiser Health News in 2014, Rabin cited evidence that provider office visits had consistently decreased in length since Medicare's 1992 shift away from "usual and customary" payments that reflected the prevailing community rates for similar services.[215] Newer reimbursement models provided a system of paying for "relative value units" (RVUs) that reflected a provider's effort and costs of running an office to determine the "actual value" of time spent in patient care. Frequently pitting health-care consumer demand for more time to have questions answered against a provider's desire to shorten office visit times to maximize revenue led to further erosion in the bond between provider and consumer. As greater use of ambulatory electronic health records began to be deployed, physicians were feeling even more time constrained, since they were given the additional task of entering data into the electronic record at the time of the patient encounter. One office-based clinical cardiologist I interviewed expressed it best on behalf of his colleagues when he said, "I spent a total of fourteen years after high school becoming proficient in the specialty of cardiology, and I find myself now nothing more than an overpaid data entry technician."[216]

In an article in *JAMA* from 1999, primary-care physicians were found to interrupt and redirect a patient's chief concern after only twenty-three seconds of starting a clinical encounter, and many patients did not get an opportunity to finalize planning for those concerns that were left unheard.[217] In a 2001

215 R. C. Rabin, "You're on the Clock: Doctors Rush Patients out the Door", Kaiser Health News in *USA Today*, April 20, 2014, accessed April 3, 2017, https://www.usatoday.com/story/news/nation/2014/04/20/doctor-visits-time-crunch-health-care/7822161/.

216 Quote attributed to Joel From, MD, clinical cardiologist, Des Moines, Iowa.

217 M. K. Marvek, "Soliciting the Patient's Agenda: Have We Improved?," *Journal of the American Medical Association* 281, no. 3 (1999): 283–287.

study of family medicine and internal medicine residents, the average length of time following entry into a patient room until that physician interrupted the conversation was twelve seconds, and during an average eleven-minute encounter, only four minutes were spent actively listening to patient issues.[218] From the same study, resident physicians were interrupted by telephone calls and computer alerts an average of two times per patient encounter, and those residents identified computer interruptions as taking the greatest amount of time away from direct patient care. Reflecting further erosion of communication channels between provider and consumer, primary-care physicians were found to address only 54.9 percent of recommended care practices for patients in their offices due to time constraints. Interviews with primary-care residency chairpersons suggested that to be fully compliant with providing all the preventive and routine medical care needed by patients in an office practice, a physician would need to be in an office setting for twenty-five hours of every workday, clearly a difficult task for even the most ambitious young health-care provider.[219] With greater degrees of time pressure felt by providers and consumers alike, it is little wonder that stress levels among clinicians have been progressively rising and provider burnout has begun to take a toll on the existing workforce and the relationship that doctors share with their patients.

In a recent report from the American Hospital Association, several hospital representatives interviewed stressed the importance of bringing "joy and meaning" back to the workplace to build resilience and to decrease burnout seen in health-care providers.[220] In the same study, it was also suggested that a renewed focus on employee wellness programs should be started and that efforts should be made to embrace comprehensive well-being of providers, establish patient and worker safety programs, and identify ways to provide environmental accommodations for an aging workforce. The committee cited

218 D. R. Rhoades et al., "Speaking and Interruptions during a Primary Care Office Visit," *Family Medicine* 33, no. 7 (2001): 528–532.

219 E. A. McGlynn et al., "The Quality of Health Care Delivered to Adults in the United States," *New England Journal of Medicine* 348 (2003): 2635–2645.

220 K. McNally et al., *The Imperative for Strategic Workforce Planning and Development: Challenges and Opportunities*, Committee on Performance Improvement, 2017, accessed April 3, 2017, http://www.aha.org/content/17/cpi-report.pdf.

several policy changes being promulgated that could produce further stresses, such as the new payment system being proposed to reimburse physicians, called the Medicare Access and CHIP Reauthorization Act (MACRA) of 2015.[221] Other financial stresses tied to reimbursement system changes include those associated with the demonstration projects that were funded under the Affordable Care Act calling for Accountable Care Organizations to focus on methods that a health system can employ to take on clinical and financial risk for providing care for large populations of patients using a capitated fee structure.[222] Such a capitated payment system rewards shortened patient visits for clinical conditions of low severity. Providers in many ways feel helpless as such financial changes directly impact their livelihood and societal standing.

These moving pieces have contributed to several new ways in which health-care providers and health-care consumers are charged with working together and learning to communicate differently. The days of a health-care provider being available twenty-four hours a day, seven days a week disappeared long ago, but one needs to wonder what the new social compact being created today will lead to in the years ahead. Despite all the advancements made technically in our ability to deliver higher-quality solutions and to capture information electronically, a great deal of dissatisfaction remains for both providers and consumers. Even with a desire to include patients and families in discussions regarding the health strategies that are based on preferences found in their intrinsic value systems, and even as providers continue their personal mission of practicing the very human science of health care, it becomes more and more difficult to do so in an environment where financial efficiency has become the driving force for many clinicians. Many providers have become disillusioned but still profess their love for a profession that they selected to help people in need. Many consumers still want and demand the

---

221 Centers for Medicare and Medicaid Services, "MACRA, Delivery System Reform, Medicare Payment Reform," accessed May 25, 2017, https://www.cms.gov/Medicare/Quality-Initiatives-Patient-Assessment-Instruments/Value-Based-Programs/MACRA-MIPS-and-APMs/MACRA-MIPS-and-APMs.html..

222 Centers for Medicare and Medicaid Services, "Accountable Care Organizations," accessed May 25, 2017, https://www.cms.gov/Medicare/Medicare-Fee-for-Service-Payment/ACO/index.html.

very best from their personal health providers at all times of the day and night, leaving clinicians but empty shells of their former selves. Health-care consumers have stepped forward to take on greater responsibility and accountability for their care decisions, but they continue to need the learned guidance from their provider partners, who are now seen less as autonomous professionals and more as equal members of a consumer's personalized health-care team. Health-care policy makers continue to make efforts to slow the rate of rise in global health-care budgets that they fear will eventually break the American piggy bank, while health-care manufacturers and pharmaceutical companies continue to design and implement better, faster, and more powerful alternatives to yesterday's medical products, devices, and medications.

In the most personal of all health-care experiences, too many conflicting agendas have led to a place where all participants are feeling unfulfilled. This new transactional space has been emptied of the joy and hope that we should expect in a country with tremendous financial resources and an entrepreneurial spirit. Perhaps innovation science may eventually help us find the crossroads of designing pristine care processes along with a rejuvenated focus on caring for and about one another. Until that time comes, we will need to be vigilant about the impact from erosion of the long-standing compact that has for years forged deep and long-lasting relationships between care providers and consumers. Most participants in this dance of life want to share this delicate interface with another human engaged in a committed and personal quest for better health. If asked whether I would rather choose a provider who is a superb technician, having attended the best medical school and residency programs in the country, or someone who was less well trained but who cares for me deeply during the times I need the person most, I would quite simply answer that I would want both.

Key Points to Master From Chapter 11

- *The AMA Code of Medical Ethics* describes the practice of medicine as a fundamentally moral activity. The clinical encounter is based on a trust-based relationship where a physician places the patients' welfare above the physicians' own self-interests or obligations to others. Patients have "the right to receive information and ask questions about recommended treatments so they can make well-considered decisions about care". Physicians are counseled that if laws or regulations are proposed that are contrary to the best interest of patients, physicians are to seek changes in those requirements to keep patients' interests at the forefront. The code calls for physicians to support access to medical care for all people.
- In 2002, the Medical Professionalism Project called for:
  o Primacy of patient welfare above all else
  o Patient autonomy and participation in decision making
  o Social justice so that care would be delivered equitably
- The 2017 Organizational Professionalism Charter Project outlined:
  o A need to develop patient partnerships as processes are designed
  o Promotion of a culture of trust and empowerment
  o Addressing social determinants of health through community collaboration and cooperation
  o Focus on cost-effective health care without conflicts of interest
- As the medical information age unfolded, consumers had expanded access to data that created a more empowered consumer; the social compact between provider and consumer had to evolve in response.
- Providers feel helpless as financial changes such as MACRA, expanding physician employment relationships, and risk-bearing ACOs have arisen, as each of these has directly impacted their livelihood and societal standing.
- Providers continue their personal mission of practicing the very human science of healthcare, but it is now more difficult to do so

when financial efficiency has become the driving force. Consumers have taken on greater responsibility and accountability for care decisions, but still need the learned guidance of provider partners who are now seen less as autonomous professionals and more as equal members of a consumer's personalized health care team.

Section 3
The Path Forward

INTRODUCTION TO SECTION 3

With so many influential voices directing the structure and function of today's health-care delivery systems, it is essential to assess the utility of the current state of health-care delivery while reflecting on the future of those systems. What is heard in conversations with health-care consumers and health-care providers alike is a general feeling of dissatisfaction with the present state, one in which moments of dynamic tension exist and where opportunities for improvement can be realized. Many new, innovative tools and methods have been uncovered or improved on since the antibiotic era ushered in tremendous improvements in life-span and quality of life. No longer is it routine to find Americans dying from common infectious diseases or from common health-care experiences such as childbirth, and these improvements must be celebrated as distinct enhancements to our way of life. The speed of rolling out these enhancements has been quite uneven, with some improvements coming at lightning speed that has exceeded the adoption comfort of providers and consumers, while other improvements have left many wondering why it has taken so long to adopt such obvious strides forward that could lead to better quality of life and health status. A great deal of finger pointing has resulted as a result, with providers complaining about adequate and fair reimbursement for their time and efforts, the federal and private payers wringing their hands over the spiraling costs of health care, and patients and families wondering whether anyone is actually caring about their perceptions of a cold and impersonal care delivery experience.

To better understand the dynamic of what is to come, we must first focus on two key issues that face health-care delivery participants today: how health care is (dis)organized and the unintended consequences of a new social compact that has been created as a result of the many voices striving to redesign the health care experience. If the foibles and blessings of the current state can be better understood, it is then possible to forecast what the future system for health-care delivery might look like. While no one has a crystal ball that will perfectly outline the care-delivery system of the future, several principles that will guide the design of that system can be discerned, and components of that care system can be outlined. The greatest desire of this guide is to stimulate all participants to cooperate and to design the new system together, so that the most innovative approaches can be used to bridge the greatest number of individual agendas, which will lead to a health-care system that will work for the greatest number of people. Since illness and injury is something that affects all Americans, it will be important to project the most likely scenarios that will come and to allow inclusive public debate around the policy issues that will most certainly drive the future delivery system in terms of relationships, funding, and outcomes. At the very heart of these debates, all parties should continue to focus on how we can all work together to save the heart of the American health-care experience.

Twelve

WHO IS RESPONSIBLE FOR TAKING CARE OF MY MOTHER?

With all the variation that occurs in the clinical presentation of human disease, it is no wonder that the systematic delivery of health care brings with it a unique set of approaches that differentiates the practice of medicine from all other enterprises. A health-care interaction centers on the methods used by a group of practitioners to favorably impact the health status of an individual afflicted with an illness or injury, and each clinical condition under evaluation can be acute or chronic, preventive or acutely interventional, and it can affect humans of any age. The resultant complexity of such interactions can make health-care system redesign quite complicated and incomplete in its formulated solutions, always leaving open the potential for improvement. To thoughtfully design for the future, it will serve care designers well to better understand the successes and challenges experienced in today's health-care delivery systems. Looking at actual care-delivery scenarios developed from a variety of care experiences in which I participated as a provider, the reader should understand better the anatomy of health-care experiences and how care redesign teams could create more effective and efficient approaches that will address tomorrow's health-care needs. The following scenarios demonstrate the spectrum of current health-care delivery services and how they are organized.

Scenario #1—Acute Medical Illness. When a person presents to a medical office, an urgent-care center, or a hospital emergency department, that person's medical affliction has generally culminated in a series of diagnostic symptoms and signs that reflect the subtle progression of an illness. Sophie G.'s case represents a simple example of such a condition, the development of acute bacterial pneumonia in which shortness of breath, productive cough, and chest pain produced enough discomfort that she sought medical care. After taking a detailed patient history, her doctor performed a routine limited examination and ordered laboratory tests and an X-ray of her chest to establish a diagnosis.

In the *asymptomatic phase* of her illness, Sophie, a sixty-three-year-old mother of three who had been in fairly good health, had remained at home with only minor symptoms that were underestimated for four days, since her symptoms were generally not very severe, and she had an aversion to medical care that was driven by her previous health-care experiences. Complicating the decision to seek medical assistance, Sophie's personal value system suggested to her that she could recover from such a minor inconvenience in her own home using the self-care recommendations that she had used in raising her own children. Weighing heavily in her decision to seek medical care was an underlying concern she had regarding her personal financial status, since she lacked health insurance coverage.

Moving into the *acute diagnostic and initial therapeutic phase* of her illness, Sophie was admitted to the hospital for intravenous fluids and antibiotics, oxygen therapy, and chest physical therapy, with monitoring by nursing staff. To meet the needs of her acute medical illnesses, Sophie was assigned to a treating provider who was a hospital-based internal medicine specialist with experience in providing care for acutely ill individuals. The doctor's roles included providing acute care, communicating with Sophie's family to coordinate a treatment plan that would be continued after her discharge from hospital, and establishing goals of her care. Orders for medications and other treatments were written by the admitting doctor, and a team that included the physician, nurse, and pulmonary therapists evaluated Sophie for any change in her clinical status to confirm that adequate medical progress toward recovery was being made. Other hospital-based treatment team members, such as dietary therapy, physical therapy, and chaplaincy services, met with Sophie to address nutritional, functional, and spiritual care needs, and pharmacists provided the needed medications to promote her recovery. A hospital case manager monitored her care progress to coordinate discharge to the most appropriate level of service, deciding between a discharge to home or to a care facility for additional rehabilitative care. At admission, and throughout the course of the hospital stay, insurance information was sought and a plan confirmed to guarantee payment for services, since medical insurance coverage was lacking. Because Sophie did not have insurance coverage, she met with the hospital's financial services representatives to establish payment terms following discharge from hospital. Information-technology services supported the electronic health record that provided therapeutic guidance for Sophie's care and established a communication channel for the care team to document pertinent findings. Hospital-based physicians, called hospitalists, rotated daily as shift workers, and they monitored Sophie's medical progress and passed along their thoughts regarding her ongoing care needs as her discharge plan was further refined.

A *transitional phase* occurred when Sophie became healthy enough for discharge, and self-care information was reviewed with her by hospital staff. Nursing personnel evaluated Sophie's ongoing care needs at home, instructed her how the care plan should be continued, and outlined her ambulatory follow-up care with an office-based clinician. After being discharged from hospital, Sophie entered the *recuperative* or *rehabilitative phase*, where her medical care was once again coordinated with her primary-care physician. If Sophie could not have performed adequate self-care at home, she might have been admitted for a brief period to rehabilitate in a skilled nursing facility, where ongoing assistance would have been provided to carry out the care plan and help her regain her independence at home.

These phases of acute medical care happen thousands of times each day across the country and are nearly flawless in their execution, but in some instances, confusion can arise in determining which clinician is named as the ultimate decision-maker. This lack of strategic approach clouds the longitudinal care plan that defines the person's ongoing needs following discharge from the hospital, muddies the timing for discharge, and does not clarify precisely the individual charged with oversight of a patient's longer-term care coordination. It is in these instances where confusion exists, the American health-care delivery system fails, and patients and their families are left to ask the question, who's in charge of my mother's care? Where confusion exists, longer-term clinical outcomes are less than stellar, and the person and family are frequently left unsatisfied as health-care consumers, questioning the overall value of the services that have been provided.

Scenario #2—Acute Surgical Care. When John Q., a fifty-four-year-old divorced man, developed acute abdominal pain after dinner, his first thoughts turned to the three-day-old leftover chicken that he had pulled from the refrigerator to eat. John took some chewable antacids, lay down on the couch to watch another rerun of *Friends*, and hoped his nausea and pain would subside on their own. In this case, the *asymptomatic phase* was absent, since he developed an acute onset of abdominal pain and nausea over a very brief period. As hours passed, his pain increased, and it began to localize to the lower left portion of his abdomen. When he began to sweat and feel feverish, he took liquid antacids and a stomach acid blocker, and he called his doctor's office. Since it was after office hours, the doctor's partner called John back after a twenty-five-minute wait. When the doctor heard of John's complaints, and since he did not have access to John's medical record, he instructed the man to go to the emergency department for the *diagnostic* and *therapeutic phase* of his acute illness. Missed in the telephone conversation was John's previous history of having had three abdominal surgeries as a result of a gunshot wound to the abdomen suffered during an after-hours altercation at a bar on the city's south side.

Despite the pain, John felt well enough to drive himself to the local hospital, where an admitting intake nurse took his medical history. Since the emergency room was packed and John did not appear to be *in extremis*, the nurse asked John to take a seat in the waiting room. After a two-hour wait, John called to the unit secretary that his pain was getting severe and asked about how much longer he would be waiting before being seen by a doctor. An hour later, John was profusely sweating, bent over at the waist due to significant pain, and vomited on the waiting room floor. He was taken quickly to an emergency evaluation area, where laboratory and X-rays revealed that he had a near-complete blockage of his small intestine, most likely from internal scar tissue from his previous surgeries. Somewhat similar to strings of spaghetti, internal scars can form following surgical or traumatic healing of wounds, and these strands can close off the bowel, producing sudden abdominal pain, fever, nausea, and vomiting, and if not treated appropriately, they can lead to rupture or perforation of the intestine that may cause overwhelming infection.

John was admitted to the hospital's surgical floor and had a tube placed through his nose into his stomach to decompress the backup of air and fluid that had accumulated behind the intestinal blockage. When he did not respond to conservative care, John was seen by a consulting surgeon, who determined that another surgical procedure would be needed to free up the scar tissue that was producing John's medical issues. Entering the *acute care phase*, John was taken to the operating room, where surgery to relieve his blockage was performed. Then he was taken to the surgical ward, where he received additional intravenous fluids and antibiotics, and the care coordination process began. He was seen most days by the surgeon's physician assistant, who coordinated the care plan, working with nursing staff and discharge planning staff to prepare John for his return home.

Following a few days of acute care after his procedure, plans were finalized to send John home with home care assistance to monitor his clinical recovery. Home care nursing staff would also make certain that he would take adequate food and fluids to regain strength and to promote healing. The *transitional plan* was completed when the discharge nurse provided education about post-discharge care and asked John to "teach back" to her what he had learned so that she could be sure that John knew what to expect following his discharge. Returning home, John cleaned out his refrigerator of all leftovers that were now two weeks old, and he *recuperated* with the assistance of a home healthcare nurse who helped coordinate John's surgical office visits.

John's case represents a few points concerning acute surgical care. When John was at home, he had little ability to engage in meaningful dialogue with a physician who knew his medical history, since the office was closed, and John's doctor was not "on call" to receive his initial cry for help. Not being able to access an office level of service, the next available logical site of service for John's evaluation was the emergency department, which in his case was probably the most appropriate place to be seen. When he arrived at the hospital emergency department, it was choked with a variety of people seeking medical care for conditions that ranged from earache to heart attack, and the triage nurse who first saw John had to use her expertise to match the available resources with the needs of all the individuals seeking acute and urgent care. John finally demonstrated a high enough degree of illness burden that he was taken to be seen by a physician, who established the diagnosis that ultimately resulted in John's admission to hospital and his surgical procedure to relieve intestinal blockage. A consulting doctor saw John and performed a technical procedure to relieve the blockage, but the surgeon was never seen again at the bedside, deferring John's care to a lesser-trained individual called a physician assistant. Most of John's care and discharge planning were carried out by nursing staff and discharge coordinators who were social workers, and his *recuperative phase* at home was monitored by a home health nurse, with very little input from a physician except for a single office visit to assess the healing of John's surgical wounds. Although he was given some educational materials regarding the home care of his surgical site, very little information was given to him about evaluation of complications from the procedure or about early recognition of symptoms that might signal a recurrence of his condition. Even less information was provided about the follow-up care he would need to address the elevated cholesterol and high blood pressure that were found during his highly focused surgical care admission.

Scenario #3—The Elective Surgical Procedure. Michael Z. was a star high-school running back who made a name for himself as a scholarship athlete at a Division II college. During his senior year, while participating in one of the many practice sessions in which he gave up his body for the good of the team, Michael twisted his right knee as he was attempting to make a spin move that would have allowed him to elude a tackler. Hearing a pop and feeling a sudden weakness and pain that caused him to fall to the ground, Michael realized that his collegiate career as a running back was suddenly coming to an end. He was offered options for care that included urgent surgery to repair three pieces of internal supporting structures within his knee, but the second option of conservative nonoperative care was far more attractive, since the thought of surgery did not appeal to him.

Now, forty-five years later, Michael's daily ritual of jogging had become nearly unbearable, with pain and swelling foiling his efforts to use copper-impregnated support sleeves that he wore on both knees to allow him to exercise. Discussing options for management with his primary-care physician, Michael opted for a surgical procedure to replace his defective knee joints, and he was referred to an orthopedic surgeon who specialized in knee replacement procedures. An educated man with a strong preference for information regarding any decision he made, Michael wanted to better understand the quality of work historically provided by the surgeon to whom he would entrust his future jogging career. He asked his primary-care doctor about the reputation of the surgeon being recommended and was told that the orthopedic surgeon had performed hundreds of these surgeries in the past, had a good reputation among his colleagues, and was affiliated with an outstanding hospital where the work would be performed. Nothing further could be deduced from the office conversation, so Michael accepted the recommendation and secured a follow-up appointment with the orthopedic physician.

While waiting three weeks for the next available appointment, Michael spoke with a friend who told him about a high degree of variability in orthopedic quality and suggested that he look into the health-care quality-reporting sites that were publicly available on the Internet. During this period of inquiry, Michael found that his orthopedic surgeon had attended a highly respected medical school and residency, had been in practice for twenty-six years, and was board certified by the American Academy of Orthopedic Surgeons, but he had been sued twice for care that had not gone as anticipated.[223] The hospital had a three-star rating from the Centers for Medicare and Medicaid Services, and information regarding their quality and safety showed that the hospital's

---

223 From UCompareHealthCare.com, one of many sites reporting on physician quality.

postoperative rates of deep vein thrombosis (clotting in the legs following surgery) were higher than expected and higher than surrounding hospitals.[224,225] Michael made a mental note of this and vowed to ask the orthopedic surgeon to help clarify these findings so that he could spend time focusing on preparing for the upcoming procedure.

During the *diagnostic phase* of Michael's care planning, he met with the orthopedic physician, had his knees examined and X-rays taken, and asked about the findings regarding the hospital's rates of clotting after surgery. The orthopedic surgeon did not advise his patient to immediately proceed to surgery, stating that "when the time was right," Michael would know when to have knee replacement surgery. Michael returned home, opened a blog to see how other people had decided about the timing of their surgical knee replacement, and even looked for second opinions regarding nonoperative care for his knee pain.[226]

After three very difficult months with increasing pain, decreased ability to run, and an increasing reliance on over-the-counter painkillers, Michael thought that this was the time that his orthopedic surgeon had highlighted as the "right time" to proceed. An appointment was made to have a presurgical medical clearance that included a complete physical exam and a review of medications, allergies, and previous medical history to ensure that no unanticipated medical conditions might be looming that would adversely affect his surgery and recuperation. The next stop was a return orthopedic appointment where he briefly saw the surgeon, but most of Michael's questions about the procedure were answered by the surgeon's office assistant. During the visit, laboratory tests were reordered since the previous results could not be immediately accessed from the primary-care doctor's office, and insurance information regarding Medicare coverage was obtained. In addition, to verify that he

224 Centers for Medicare and Medicaid Services, "Physician Compare," accessed May 25, 2017, https://www.medicare.gov/physiciancompare/#search.

225 Centers for Medicare and Medicaid Services, "Hospital Compare," accessed May 25, 2017, https://www.cms.gov/Medicare/Quality-Initiatives-Patient-Assessment-Instruments/Hospital QualityInits/HospitalCompare.html.

226 E. Carey, "The Best Knee Replacement Blogs of the Year," *Healthline*, May 6, 2014, accessed May 25, 2017, http://www.healthline.com/health-slideshow/best-total-knee-replacement-blogs#2.

was aware and informed of the decision to proceed with a knee replacement, Michael participated in review of a decision aid that helped frame a conversation around the alternatives to surgery, the risks and benefits of surgical treatment, and finalizing a specific course of action that was consistent with his value system. This process, called "shared decision-making," has been written about extensively[227] and promotes a facilitated discussion that helps an individual guide the treatment plan based on meaningful and tailored information. While many offices and hospitals believe they provide tools to help patients to guide the decisions being made about their health,[228] most of these decision aids are ineffective in their efforts to extract patient values-driven preferences. Shared decision-making is meant to bring out the best in a provider's role as an expert in clinical evidence while recognizing that patients are the utmost expert in expressing what is most important to them.

Arriving very early at the hospital for his surgical date, Michael was seen by a preoperative nurse who documented that all appropriate consents for surgery were obtained and verified, that Michael had not eaten anything after midnight to help prevent anesthesia complications, and that he had not taken his routine medications, especially the daily aspirin that he had been requested to stop three days before the surgery. In the preoperative staging area, Michael saw his orthopedic surgeon, and a verification step was taken to mark the knee on which surgery was to be done to prevent a wrong-side surgery error. Then the patient met the anesthesiologist who would be responsible for making sure that Michael had his medical conditions appropriately monitored while he was undergoing the knee replacement.

When Michael awoke following the procedure, he was disoriented and confused, but he was also surrounded by a team of nurses who attended to his pain and who provided comforting words about how well he had done. Following his recovery from anesthesia, Michael was transferred to the orthopedic floor, where he met with the *recuperative care* team that included nursing

---

227 E. S. Spatz, H. M. Krumholz, and B. W. Moulton, "Prime Time for Hard Decision Making," *Journal of the American Medical Association* 317, no. 13 (2017).

228 J. Herrin et al., "Patient and Family Engagement: A Survey of U.S. Hospital Practices," *British Medical Journal of Quality and Safety* 25, no. 3: 182–189.

staff, a physical therapist, the care coordinator, and a dietician. He was encouraged to breathe deeply and cough frequently to prevent any segmental collapse of lung tissue that could result in pneumonia, and he was placed in bed with support stockings that came up to his midthigh to reduce postoperative clotting in his leg veins. Uncomfortable and itchy, Michael asked when the stockings could be removed, and when he was told that their purpose was to reduce the likelihood of clots forming in his legs, he was relieved that the hospital was watching for leg blood clots. Remembering that this was an important finding in the government's reporting website for this hospital, Michael elected to put up with the discomfort of the leggings so that he would not suffer a known complication of this procedure.

After a few days, Michael could negotiate the hospital walking paths with assistance, and care coordinators helped plan Michael's discharge to a care facility where he would more thoroughly focus on his mobility and knee functional status. His medical conditions were stable, and he was once again on a daily aspirin as he had been before admission. On day three of the skilled nursing home stay, Michael's right leg began to swell considerably, and he had a painful cord that he could feel under his skin just above the knee that had been repaired. The skilled facility's nursing staff conferred with the doctor who was making rounds that day, and the suspicion was that Michael had suffered a postoperative complication of a clotted blood vessel related to his surgery. When the operating doctor was called, Michael was transferred back to a different hospital to have his clots treated with intravenous blood thinners. Only much later did Michael find out that his blood-clotting episode would not be reported on the government's quality website, since the complication had occurred in one hospital but had been treated in another hospital, thereby absolving the original surgical institution of any obligation to report to the government website. Michael just wanted to get well, return home, and get about the business of living a better quality of life without pain and certainly without a clot in his leg. After six weeks of care in the skilled facility and at home, Michael was well enough to begin going for brief walks without the pain he had previously experienced, but with significant weakness and stiffness of the affected knee that had been replaced. It took Michael nearly four months to gain enough strength and mobility to even consider resuming his habit of jogging, and he was certain that he would defer any surgery on the other knee for fear of losing four to six more months of fair health by having a repeat of the experience he had just completed.

Scenario #4—Preventive Care. Rory was a seventeen-year-old senior high-school student preparing for his first foray in freedom when he would enter as a freshman at a prominent university. Always in good health, he was perpetually in the *asymptomatic phase* and was beginning the process of transferring his care from his lifelong pediatrician, searching for an internal medicine doctor who would assume his ongoing medical care. As part of his fall enrollment in college, Rory needed a complete physical examination and a variety of immunizations to make certain that he remained healthy while residing in an institutionalized college dormitory setting. His mother set an appointment date for late summer, having first called the new practitioner's office in early April. Elective physical exams were a relatively low priority for the office, especially since the loss of one of the practice site physicians had left the remaining three doctors overworked and with few openings. Rory's pediatrician had office records that were computerized when the office shifted from paper charts to an electronic health record, and most of his previous office encounters had been scanned into the computer. Since his new doctor was using a different electronic medical record, Rory's mother requested that his previous medical records be printed out, and, after driving to the office and paying a twenty-five-dollar fee for copying, she personally carried the records to Rory's new doctor's office. Most of the record was complete, but missing was the report of a misadventure at the beach, when Rory had slipped on some rocks and suffered a facial laceration that was repaired at a local hospital emergency department. Also missing was a visit to the local Walgreen's pharmacy where he had received an influenza vaccination the year before, but since Rory's health had been otherwise excellent, these deficiencies in documentation seemed of little importance.

Following a routine history and physical examination and with no laboratory or X-ray studies performed, Rory completed the *diagnostic phase* of his health experience and was declared to be fit and ready for college the following month. As part of the *therapeutic phase* of his health-care transaction, Rory was offered a vaccination against meningitis, which was recommended for all incoming college freshmen, and he was reminded to get a flu shot when on campus. Due to time limitations in the office, the provider deferred discussions about alcohol and drug use, sexual health habits and preferences, risks of tobacco use, stress management and preventive behavioral health care, and dietary counseling. A series of immunizations for HPV, a common and preventable cancer-producing virus that can be transmitted through sexual contact, was not offered.

As Rory left for the university, his parents reminded him to register for student health services and to get a flu shot in the late fall. Most of the rest of Rory's health education would have to come from his fellow dorm residents and from materials that were distributed through the dormitories regarding sexually transmitted diseases and the perils of drug use. A condom dispenser was located in the dormitory's first-floor bathroom, providing a reminder to Rory and his friends of the importance of preventing sexual disease transmission. After the second weekend of the first semester, when a freshman student was taken by ambulance to the local emergency department after suffering injuries from a fall that was related to excess alcohol consumption, Rory's resident advisor held an information session with the students on his floor to remind each of them about the university's prohibition against drinking on campus, reinforcing the hazards of drinking to excess.

From this scenario, one can see that health information is frequently received piecemeal and in informal settings. While parents hope that their offspring are safe and careful while away at college, no unifying strategy for comprehensively educating about health risks for college students is currently being promoted. Rory received several bits of preventive health information from a variety of sources that included his physician, his parents, his dormitory staff, his fellow students, and the Internet, but the quality of this information could not be assured, making his health journey quite fragmented.

Scenario #5—Obstetrical Care and Neonatal Intensive Care. Julie was ecstatic when she saw the results from the home pregnancy test confirming what she already knew, that her first baby would arrive in approximately seven short months. From her previous networking and a check of her insurance provider network status, Julie had already picked out the obstetrical practice she wanted to use for her delivery. Shifting quickly through the *asymptomatic phase* of her health-care experience, through the *diagnostic phase*, and immediately into the *acute care phase*, Julie was giddy as she arrived at her initial appointment with the obstetrician. Blood and urine tests were performed, looking for early signs of maternal diabetes or genetic abnormalities in the baby, and additional screening studies were performed for clinical conditions that might affect the mother's and baby's health during pregnancy. Measurements of the uterine height were done, blood pressure was screened, and an ultrasound of the pregnancy was requested. This standardized, full-service approach had been evolving over many years, but its essential core testing approach was initially designed to give assurance to both the mother and the provider team that the "products of conception" were safe and stable so that the pregnancy would have the highest likelihood for success.

Julie and her husband were simultaneously thrilled and concerned when they were told that Julie's pregnancy would bring them the special gift of twins. Monthly follow-up visits to the office demonstrated satisfactory progress with growth of the twin boys at acceptable rates and no evidence of complications such as high blood pressure or diabetes, and all genetic screening tests returned normal. It was not until late in the twenty-fifth week that a small amount of vaginal bleeding caused Julie to phone the OB office for instructions. An appointment was made for that day, and after the visit revealed nothing unusual, Julie was instructed to remain at complete bed rest at home and to phone the office day or night should anything unusual arise such as cramping, contractions, or further bleeding. For nearly a week, Julie dutifully stayed in bed, and her husband doted over her every need, even asking for assistance from Julie's mother to attend to daytime needs when he was at work.

In the middle of the twenty-sixth week of pregnancy, contractions began, and following a telephone check-in with her obstetrician's office, Julie was instructed to proceed to the hospital to be evaluated, entering a secondary *diagnostic* and *therapeutic phase* of her health-care experience. An initial assessment of Julie's pregnancy was completed, and efforts were made to slow and stop her uterine contractions. After an initial success, the contractions became unstoppable, and Julie delivered two boys, one weighing two pounds three ounces and the second just a bit over two pounds. The newborns were transferred to the hospital's neonatal intensive care unit (NICU), where they required breathing assistance using a ventilator, and they had intravenous lines inserted through an umbilical blood vessel so that medications and monitoring could be performed. Every horror story that Julie had ever heard raced through her mind, and she wondered aloud to her husband whether they would ever become the complete and happy family that they had envisioned when they first heard the news of their pregnancy.

As the days moved forward, Julie was discharged from the hospital to begin her personal *recuperative phase*, while the boys were just beginning their *acute care* journey with a rude awakening of what life could bring. Slowly but steadily, the boys turned the corner, and after their initial breathing difficulties were stabilized, they were *transitioned* to a less intensive portion of the NICU where they could "feed and grow" in anticipation of being discharged to their new home. Not many years previously, common medical knowledge held that a child born at twenty-six weeks was "nonviable," and efforts at keeping a child comfortable while awaiting his or her inevitable passage were all that could be offered. In 2016, Julie's boys had the full benefit of recent advances in ventilator technology, new medications to help keep their lungs expanded and exchanging oxygen, monitoring devices that could identify the earliest changes in a newborn's clinical status, and new research that could help determine the precise level of oxygen that would support each child's development while avoiding the toxic state of too much oxygen that could result in damage to their eyes.

Just seven and a half weeks after their premature arrival, Julie and her husband *transitioned* their new family yet again, this time to home with close follow-up with a pediatrician's office that specialized in care for premature newborns. The two boys were carefully monitored at home with close attention paid to their feeding habits, growth, and weight changes, and special attention given to treating complications early and receiving necessary vaccinations to prevent a respiratory virus that could attack them during the winter months. The *recuperative phase* for the boys was extremely successful, and when they reached a true age of premature birth plus twelve weeks, they appeared to have hit every major developmental milestone that had been outlined for them by their pediatrician. Julie, her husband, and two healthy boys had experienced the miracle of what was the best in American health care. This scenario demonstrates the high-value outcomes that can be experienced from American health-care practices that have been standardized, evidence-based, and highly integrated. With access to the latest technology and well-designed care practices, great strides have been made in the care of premature newborns.

Scenario # 6—Congestive Heart Failure as a Chronic Care Condition. A very common clinical condition for an aging population is congestive heart failure, most commonly as result of latent disease involving the small and larger arteries that supply blood to the heart muscle. The *asymptomatic phase* of disease progresses for years, as elevations in blood pressure, lack of exercise, and elevation of cholesterol related to poor dietary choices take a slow but steady toll in narrowing these blood vessels to a point where the heart muscle becomes starved for oxygen. Murray was such a person, with a diet rich in red meats, job stresses that were very high, and obesity resultant from poor diet and lack of regular aerobic exercise. Murray kept a routine annual physical examination on his calendar, and most years he was able to keep the appointment with his doctor when he wasn't out of the country traveling for business. During this *asymptomatic phase* of his congestive heart failure, Murray was instructed by his doctor that he should exercise more and eat better, and they should "talk about" starting medicines for mildly elevated blood pressure and significantly elevated cholesterol levels. Murray agreed in principle but always deferred further diagnostic testing or treatment since he felt relatively well, aside from some wheezing and shortness of breath he periodically experienced when rushing to catch a plane for a business trip.

While in San Francisco for a new client meeting, Murray awakened in the middle of the night with shortness of breath and a tightness in his chest that felt very uncomfortable. Thinking that he had been under a lot of stress and just needed to relax more, Murray tried getting back to sleep, but he found that his breathing was significantly hampered, and he was unable to lie flat in bed. By four in the morning, Murray realized that he was not going to be able to sleep and thought it might be wise to be seen in the hospital emergency department that was close to his downtown hotel. By the time Murray arrived by taxi to the hospital, he was laboring to catch his breath, and when he was seen at the front triage desk, Murray was rushed to a room where his *diagnostic phase* revealed a heart attack in evolution, and his *therapeutic phase* was immediately started. The emergency room nurse had already phoned the cardiac catheterization laboratory, and Murray was rushed to have a specialized study of his blood vessels that demonstrated nearly complete blockage of the main artery that travels down the front of the heart, a so-called "widow-maker" that, if left untreated, would probably have proved fatal.

Following several harrowing hours where balloon dilatations of Murray's arteries were performed and special drug-eluding stents were placed to keep the vessels open and reduce the likelihood of inflammation producing further narrowing and damage, Murray was *transitioned* to the cardiac care unit, where he would begin the steady progress of cardiac *rehabilitative* care. Reflecting on the many ways that he could have interceded as his own best advocate and how he and his doctor had accomplished very little to prevent his heart from injury, Murray became angry with himself and with "the system" that he perceived had failed him by not being emphatic enough to stimulate him to act. During his hospital *acute care phase*, Murray's treatment team used clinically standardized protocols to prescribe medications for blood pressure and elevated cholesterol, provide advice on how Murray could advance his exercise routine based on his tolerance, and started making plans for longer-term care planning. The care plan was coordinated by a hospital case manager, working with the cardiologists and cardiac nurses to better engage Murray in future self-care, and the team connected with a care management team in Murray's hometown, where he could continue his *recuperation phase.*

As he regained strength and made efforts to promote better conditioning, Murray was discharged home, but he noticed that despite all his best efforts, he was still quite winded when he walked, even for short distances. Now under the care of a cardiologist in his hometown, Murray had a cardiac study that showed that his heart was still quite weak, functioning poorly enough that only 15 percent of the blood in his main pumping chamber was being ejected with each heartbeat as opposed to the 55–65 percent seen normally in men his age. Because of his congestive heart failure following the acute injury to his heart, Murray was enrolled in a disease-management protocol that focused on a diverse set of medications designed to reduce the work that his heart needed to expend with each heartbeat, as well as specific education about diet, exercise, and medications. He was also given a scale to monitor his weight every day. If his weight rose more than three pounds in one day, he was to increase his water-pill dose to help shed excess fluid from his heart and lungs, and if his weight fell by more than three pounds, he was instructed to abstain from taking the water pills that day. Murray was educated about how to monitor his heart failure symptoms and when to connect with the disease manager's office for adjustments in his long-term care plan, but the goal, he was told, was for him to take control of his disease. No longer could Murray absolve himself of his duty to take responsibility for his body's health, and he was reminded that there was a team of caregivers that was committed to supporting him as long as he was willing to serve as "the captain of the ship" of his own health care.

As Murray began to get more comfortable with his congestive heart failure treatment plan, he became an advocate not only for himself, but for others suffering from the same condition. Murray began to volunteer at the hospital by providing firsthand experience to hundreds of people who were initially uncertain of their abilities to steer their own health-care decisions. Now three years removed from his "San Francisco experience," as he calls it, Murray has been able to slowly return to part-time work, and he has modified his diet and exercise to maximize the potential of his injured heart.

Scenario #7—Hospice and Palliative Care. When Vickie first heard the words "you have cancer," she had just awakened from a dreamlike state following a colonoscopy that had been performed to assess gastrointestinal bleeding. A fifty-seven-year-old divorced mother of two, Julie had a strong family history of colon cancer with a grandmother, an older sister, and an aunt who had been previously diagnosed with the condition. When holiday discussions about her family centered on how each of her deceased family members was missed, the conversation inevitably turned to how all her relatives had been on high alert for early warning signs of cancer and their adherence to colon cancer screening. The other members of her immediate family tried to help Vickie appreciate the importance of getting a screening colonoscopy performed given their family history, but she deferred, in part because she did not have health insurance. Vickie had previously held health insurance coverage as part of her work as a line worker in a small manufacturing company until their doors were shuttered during the great recession of 2007. Laid off at a time when employment was difficult to secure, Vickie took two part-time jobs to help manage the financial challenges of being the primary bread-winner for her family. There were rumors that a new government-sponsored health plan was in the offing under President Obama, but at the time when Vickie first experienced bleeding, she could only hope that it would cease on its own and that she could return to her normal life. When her bleeding became even more profuse, she was worried that she would need to see a doctor and hoped that it would not prove to be the same condition that had plagued other members of her family.

Following the colonoscopy, however, her worst nightmares had come true, and she listened carefully as the gastroenterologist told her what would occur next during her journey through a *diagnostic and therapeutic* care experience. X-rays, blood tests, and additional appointments all added to her stress, since she was reminded at each visit that financial arrangements would be needed to pay for the medical expenses that she would incur. Vickie's best choice was to secure her appointments through the local county hospital clinics, but she still worried that her family would be strapped with medical bills that could not be paid. The evaluation of her colon cancer progressed slowly, since open appointments for clinic visits were limited, and there was also a significant backlog in the X-ray department.

After a few weeks, she met with her county health clinic doctor, who reviewed the findings with her, confirming that she had a very late-stage colon cancer that would not benefit from surgery, and she would also not likely benefit from chemotherapy. As her therapeutic options appeared to be quite limited, she turned the conversation to the next steps of her *therapeutic phase* and asked about how she could get the most out of her remaining days, since she had previously experienced the agonizing struggle of several of her family members as they succumbed to their illness. Although her doctor was not fully familiar with services that were available to Vickie at this phase of her illness, he did provide a referral to the palliative care clinic, where Vickie met with a team of clinicians who were specially trained to help those who were struggling with decisions at the end of their lives. Palliative care, she was told, was specifically for people with serious or life-threatening conditions who wanted to focus on attaining the highest possible quality of life following a recognition that more intensive individualized care was not likely to produce a cure. Designed to address the emotional, physical, and spiritual issues that arise when one faces such a serious condition, palliative care is delivered in a culturally sensitive manner that reflects a person's preferences based on their value system, focusing on the most important health outcomes as defined by a person and their family members. Rather than measuring success by the simple metric of whether a person lives or dies from more intensive treatment plans, palliative care is primarily designed to maximize the value found in every day lived, helping afflicted individuals appreciate the time that they are given and how they can be more intentional spending those days.

As Vickie became more engaged with her palliative care team, she realized that they would serve as her guides along a journey that was very well-known to them, even if it was still a mystery to her. The palliative care team provided medications for pain and anxiety, made certain that Vickie's nutritional needs were addressed, and even connected Vickie with her church, a place she had not been for more than ten years. Solutions were developed that would help her children find stability in living with other family members following Vickie's passing, and a new sense of "wholeness" began creeping into her daily life. As the colon cancer progressed and Vickie developed tumors in her brain that clouded her thinking and left her sleepy for extended periods of every day, the hospice team supported Vickie at home until the end of her life, where she passed peacefully.

For Vickie, where the health-care system had initially failed her given her lack of insurance coverage, the best and most compassionate parts of the health-care system were present when she needed them most. Her personalized *transition phase* of a health-care experience was one in which she felt supported and in community with her family to the moment when she took her final breath. As difficult as it is to say good-bye to a friend or family member who succumbs to a fatal disease, it should be recognized that this health-care experience is one of the most important to health-care providers and consumers, and it should be the focal point where the social compact between the parties should be the strongest and most intentional in its execution. From a Kaiser Family Foundation Tracking Poll, 89 percent of respondents felt that compassionate care at the end of life was a very important part of a physician-patient relationship, but only 83 percent responded that their physician had ever held such a conversation with them.[229]

Aside from holding discussions about end-of-life care with a spouse, health-care providers were identified as the people with whom the greatest degree of comfort should be experienced in holding such discussions. Most respondents felt that the time needed to hold these important conversations should be reimbursed by Medicare (81 percent responded that services should be covered) and private insurers (83 percent responded favorably concerning coverage). From a separate survey assessing physician perceptions, 99 percent of doctors felt that it was important to hold advanced-care planning conversations with their patients, but only 29 percent stated that their practices had a formal approach for holding such discussions.[230] Nearly one-third of those polled stated that they had never received formal training on how to hold conversations about death and dying with their patients, and respondents felt challenged by the uncertainty about how to initiate these conversations and the timing for them.

Not only do patients have a favorable perception of care that is delivered comprehensively and includes them and their family in key decisions being

229 B. DiJulio, J. Firth, and M. Brodie, "Kaiser Family Foundation Tracking Poll," September30, 2015, accessed May 15, 2017, http://kff.org/health-costs/poll-finding/kaiser-health-tracking-poll-september-2015/.
230 PerryUndem Research/Communication conducted for the John A. Hartford Foundation, Cambia Health Foundation, and California HealthCare Foundation, *Physicians' Views toward Advanced Care Planning and End-of-Life Conversations*, April 2016.

made, such as end-of-life care planning, but several benefits accrue to the provider as well. Results suggest that when conversations about palliative and hospice care are held with those approaching the end of their lives, 17 percent fewer hospital admissions result, 25 percent fewer invasive procedures are performed, and many fewer days are spent in intensive care units, resulting in $9,000 less spent on average health-care expenditures in the last year of a person's life.[231] Despite these humanistic and economic benefits, only 60 percent of eligible patients from the same study were referred for hospice care services, and many of those referrals came quite late in the care planning process. The skills needed to participate in end-of-life care discussions are some of the most important needed by health-care providers, but they are also a skill set that is poorly appreciated in terms of impact. Not only do these conversations favorably impact federal program budgets, but they also bring health-care consumers and health-care providers closer in relationship. Central to a provider's core mission to relieve pain and suffering, conversations with patients and families concerning the transition to the final phase of life are paramount to preserving the last vestiges of the social compact that both parties so desperately want to maintain.

Clearly, health-care experiences come through a wide array of channels and situations, but each can be broken down into phases that, when approached strategically, can yield outstanding clinical outcomes. These outcomes can result in preventing disease with a focus on wellness, treating acute medical or surgical conditions, designing a customized treatment plan for a person with chronic illness, or assisting individuals as they approach the end of their lives. The most important lesson from dealing with these conditions as they progress through these phases is to preserve the human dignity of an individual and to recognize the values that drive decisions. Promoting the strong bond and relationship between one who delivers care and one who receives it should remain as a central focus for all parties. Perhaps no other experience is as intensely personal as a health-care experience, and certainly no other experience is more

---

231 Z. Obermeyer et al., "Association between the Medicare Hospice Benefit and Health Care Utilization and Costs with Poor-Prognosis Cancer," *Journal of the American Medical Association* 312, no. 18 (2014).

rewarding to the participants. By remaining engaged in designing health-care experiences that preserve and promote this provider-consumer bond, joy from delivering on his or her personal mission can be found in health-care providers, and activated and engaged health-care consumers can feel more involved in their own life stories.

Key Points to Master From Chapter 12

- There are five key phases of illness and injury that help clarify a health care consumer's journey through a health care experience:
  - o The Asymptomatic Phase where baseline health status begins
  - o The Diagnostic Phase where symptoms and signs are evaluated
  - o The Therapeutic Phase where treatment of injury or illness occurs
  - o The Transitional Phase where shifts in care intensity are implemented
  - o The Recuperative Phase where a return to a new health baseline occurs
- Multiple Scenarios are discussed in this chapter that demonstrate the phases of the health care journey and experience.
- Greater amounts of information now exist regarding health care provider quality and the disorders that providers treat, reducing the historic information asymmetry that created an imperfect marketplace for health care consumers.
- Care planning is often highly disjointed, making it difficult to determine the care provider who is in charge of a person's plan at any one moment in a health care experience. Preventive health strategies are often incomplete and health care consumers typically hold responsibility for fulfilling preventive care plans.
- Health care consumers have become much more engaged as participants in the creation of their own care plans; some even actively lead their own care teams.

Thirteen

Unintended Consequences of
a New Social Compact

It would be difficult to argue against the preferences expressed by both health-care providers and consumers to maintain the strong bond between them, but without intending to do so, many counterbalancing forces have helped erode this bond. This country has been left with a health-care system that is more focused on efficiently delivering health-care *transactions* than on promoting the *caring* that has historically been associated with high-quality health care. But is a preference for the special bond between consumer and provider important enough for this intimate dyad to fight for as health-care finance reform policies are being entertained in Washington, DC? What keeps this dyad from imposing the will of the people by insisting that health-care service delivery should not be just transactional in nature, commoditized much like purchasing a bag of sugar or a pair of jeans? Is there anything that we can do today to have our voices heard by those who are making key decisions about the health-care services on which we rely so strongly? Is it even important enough to invest the energy into a struggle to maintain this unique and powerful bond to sustain a personal health-care experience, or are we destined to see this bond erode to an unrecognizable state, relegated to the same fate as rotary dial telephones and typewriters?

From forty years of discussions with my patients and my colleagues, I have learned that the greatest satisfaction with the health-care experience is realized when both parties conspire to accomplish something far greater than what either can do in isolation. When health-care providers approach a care experience with a font of information that is to be shared with a willing and deeply engaged consumer of care services, both parties are left with clearly established goals, a specific diagnostic and therapeutic plan, and a higher likelihood of a successful outcome as defined by the person who is most invested in that experience, the care consumer. When providers approach the delivery of health-care services as a shared experience with an activated consumer and see the delivery of a care experience as a privilege, greater joy is also realized by both parties.

The environment surrounding providers and consumers of care has changed slowly over time, much like sands shifting beneath a person's feet as they walk hand in hand along a windswept beach. These changes have affected nearly every health-care provider and consumer, giving rise to a new movement toward a multitier delivery system that includes "concierge medical practices" that provide special attention to the more personalized care needs of an individual for an additional cost not covered by traditional health insurance. Health-care providers have succumbed to this new environmental imbalance by approaching their workday as shift workers participating in a more limited care experience tailored by their selection of medical and surgical subspecialties as career paths. Just as in W. T. Sedgwick's famous experiment on watching the response of a frog to slow elevations in temperature toward boiling,[232] health-care providers and consumers have been immersed in such a slow environmental erosion of their social compact that neither party has stopped to evaluate the impact seen from the many unintended consequences that have arisen.

Impact on the health-care consumer. As health-care consumers have become more active in their care plan design, an emerging degree of empower-

---

232 W. T. Sedgwick, "On Variations of Reflex-Excitability in the Frog, Induced by Changes in Temperature," *Studies from the Biological Laboratory, Volume II,* ed. Newell Martin (Baltimore: Johns Hopkins University, 1888), accessed April 20, 2017.

ment in the traditional role of "patient" has arisen, and it has been quite valuable and personally satisfying. By reaching out to the World Wide Web, care consumers can now access resources that help them become better partners in their own health experience, and they are now much more capable of arming themselves with knowledge to better express their personal values-driven preferences. When medical literature reveals no clear-cut choice between two therapeutic options, a person's values help drive decisions that are more rewarding since the final choice of therapies rests in large part with the health-care consumer. When medication side effects arise, it is the consumer who can best identify the early side effects from a prescribed medication. This new awareness makes it easier to discuss the pros and cons of switching to a different treatment option with the provider, working together to monitor for future side effects, and keeping prescribers apprised of their patient's tolerance to the new medication.

Although this new role for health-care consumers is generally well accepted by most providers, some studies have suggested that the quality of the patient-doctor relationship might be adversely affected.[233] Consumerism may present unique challenges that can be magnified during an already rushed office appointment visit, and since behavioral psychology suggests that people are anchored to their first opinion or option, they may discount a provider's opinion should it clash with that found in research they conducted using outside resources.[234] This may be magnified further when equivalent probabilities of benefit or multidimensional choices are present that may generate more potential options, and this may further strain the discussion between provider and consumer. When conflicts between viewpoints exist, adherence to therapy can be compromised, mutual frustration can result, and trust can be eroded.

Even with these caveats, when greater amounts of information are made available to all parties, the resulting relationship can become even more strongly aligned between the consumer and the provider. The economic principle of

---

233 R. Zeckhauser and B. Sommers, "Consumerism in Health Care: Challenges and Opportunities," *American Medical Association Journal of Ethics* 15, no. 11 (2013): 988–992.

234 H. C. Sox et al., *Medical Decision Making* (Boston: Butterworth-Heinemann, a division of Reed Publishing, 1988).

the "principal-agent" relationship reflects a benefit that can be seen when both the "principal" (the health-care consumer) and the "agent" (the care provider) have a shared mental model that focuses on how best to enhance an individual's health status.[235] This relationship can lead to more effective clinical outcomes when the principal is highly activated and informed, since that person has a more deeply vested interest in his or her own health due to the personal implications of decisions affecting diagnosis or therapy. When the agent is interested in embracing a care consumer's research on a medical condition, providers can fulfill the role of a medical information clearinghouse, with more comprehensive solutions formulated and the health-care consumer's preferences realized.

Most Americans who have embraced the new role of health-care consumerism have also become more active political participants as they respond to the health-care proposals arising on Capitol Hill, such as the intensity of comment being seen in town hall meetings held to discuss the implications of the Affordable Care Act and the American Health Care Act. In congressional districts across the country, groups of average Americans have stood up to have their voices heard so that their representatives will take the true pulse of their constituents. From a survey conducted just before Donald Trump's inauguration, 76 percent of respondents stated that they were either somewhat aware or fairly well informed about changes in health-care financing that had occurred as a result of the implementation of "Obamacare," and most had opinions, either strongly favorable or strongly unfavorable, about the policies that were implemented in 2010.[236] Of those surveyed, 89 percent saw the removal of preexisting conditions as a significant favorable result of the ACA, while 74 percent cited expanded access as a key strength of the plan. In the same survey, 71 percent favored the bill's provision that allowed children under age twenty-six to remain on their parent's health plan. On the other hand, 65 percent of those polled were disappointed that the plan had raised

235 J. Green, "What Is a Principal-Agent Relationship?," accessed May 27, 2017, http://small-business.chron.com/principalagent-relationship-32117.html.
236 K. P. Anderson, "A Survey on the Impact of Health Finance Reform on Consumers and Providers," Survey Monkey, January 19, 2017.

the total cost of health premiums, while 32 percent were somewhat confused by the complicated nature of some of the aspects of the plan. In addition, 25 percent of respondents cited the implementation of individual mandates needed to generate broad risk pools to spread insurance risk as a weakness, citing the negative impact on personal liberties resulting from such individual insurance mandates.

While the overall impact of the ACA was not able to be determined by most respondents given the relatively brief time since its implementation, about half of those who did have an opinion believed that the new plan would improve quality while reducing overall health-care spending. About a third of those who responded with an opinion about the overall impact of the ACA stated that they anticipated that there would be little or no change in quality or cost from its implementation, but many stated that it was still too early to assess the longer-term impact of the plan. In general, most Americans participating in the survey felt that health care was still too expensive overall, but they stated that the current US health-care financing plan was more likely to produce better clinical outcomes than a single-payer plan such as that found in Canada.

The greatest concerns expressed by survey respondents centered on the rising cost of health-care premiums that have been experienced because of the impact of the ACA on the insurance markets, with secondary concerns tied to the spiraling costs of pharmaceuticals and hospital services. Half of the respondents wanted "something better" but were unsure what that might be, and 20 percent expressed a preference for repeal of the ACA and adoption of a free-market solution. Nearly identical to those preferring a free-market solution was the number of survey respondents who favored adoption of a single-payer federal solution. From these results, it appears that American consumers want to be better informed, and many have strongly held opinions, but there appears to be no concordance on a single solution that could be embraced by all.

Impact on the health-care provider. As the number of health-care providers is expected to shrink with the large population of baby-boomer clinicians approaching retirement age, the probability is quite high that the provider-consumer social compact will continue to evolve. Many physicians trained between 1950 and 1980 are actively considering retirement, although one in four practicing physicians are now older than the traditional retirement age of sixty-five.[237] Although many physicians in this age group report concerns about their clinical performance and academic competency regarding specific advancements in their specialty field, there remains great variation in physician quality that is not specifically tied to aging. Despite the risk for cognitive decline that comes with age, data supports that senior physicians may possess certain positive attributes that are tied to the development of a strong provider-consumer bond, such as compassion and resilience during stressful events.[238] Physicians trained since the early 1990s have experienced at least some formal training in the science of interprofessional socialization, which reinforces the importance of collaborating with all members of a treatment team, and they frequently incorporate the values-driven viewpoints of those seeking care.

The potential negative impact on the social compact can be magnified by several factors that affect nearly all health-care providers operating under the current construct. The first is related to the erosion of trust that is experienced by a provider who is approached by an activated health-care consumer with a great deal of medical information during an office visit. With time constraints and a variety of potential diagnostic and therapeutic choices presented from Internet sites that reflect variable reputability, providers can become frustrated with a consumer's request to interpret medical information. One physician I interviewed told me of a patient who occasionally brought one hundred or more pages of printed materials that had been accessed from the Internet with a request for the physician to read, interpret, and recommend treatment options based on this information.

From a recent study published by the Mayo Clinic, approximately 30 percent of practicing physicians are experiencing some form of burnout, and

---

237 W. Levinson and S. Ginsburg, "JAMA Professionalism: Is It Time to Retire?," *Journal of the American Medical Association* 317, no. 15 (2017): 1570–1571.
238 Ibid.

of those expressing this negative psychological view of their practice, only a third stated that they would choose the health-care profession if they faced that decision today.[239] When physicians begin to experience erosion in their sense that medicine is a calling, there are adverse consequences not only to the providers but to those for whom they provide care.[240] This reinforces the fact that health-care providers often begin a career with ideals that are formulated from a personal mission centered on benevolence, compassion, and promotion of the well-being of another over themselves. With a new workforce and evolving financial arrangements, many providers have begun to lose their personal mission and the human characteristics that are attached to the profession's calling. As health-care systems become larger and begin to consolidate care delivery teams, roles are frequently re-envisioned, with corporate structures that diminish the individual professionalism that most health-care providers initially exhibit and strongly favor. Complex reimbursement formulae that stress the importance of productivity lead many providers to change their practice habits to maximize production at the expense of time spent with patients. Regulatory policies, management of clinical conditions by excessively standardized treatment pathways, and public reporting of care processes and outcomes divert attention and time from some health-care providers. With the advent of the electronic health record, many providers feel that the computer has become the "patient," and the most essential role of the individual practitioner more closely approximates a medical record entry technician. More intensive specialization, in response to growing medical complexity and technical evolution, has created a group of health-care providers who frequently may not be able to put together a fully integrated care plan, and shift work in specialized areas such as hospital-based medical specialties has begun to create a group of clinicians who infrequently experience the full spectrum of a patient's clinical trajectory toward health. Ambulatory specialization, particularly of primary care, has created a group of clinicians who are well versed

---

239 T. M. Smith, *AMA Wire*, March 3, 2017, accessed March 5, 2017.

240 A. J. Jager et al., "Association between Physician Burnout and Identification with Medicine as a Calling," *Mayo Clinic Proceedings* 92, no. 3 (2017): 415–422.

in taking care of relatively simple conditions but who may lack the ability to manage more complex clinical conditions seen in hospitalized patients.

In a recent interview with Jane R., a charge nurse in her late twenties working as a management nurse in a large, urban health system that is routinely recognized for its outstanding clinical outcomes, she told me that while she continues to find her chosen profession stimulating and energizing on most days, there are some days when she and her fellow nurses leave the facility barely able to walk given the fatigue from the sheer volume of work. Jane became interested in nursing by watching the care and compassion that her mother gave to her patients as a registered nurse, and she believed that the personal rewards that her mother experienced in providing care for those most in need would be the same rewards she would find when she started her own career. As operational stresses have increased and workloads have become unpredictable barriers to reasonable work-life balance, it is not surprising that what Jane experiences is not exactly what she hoped to find based on the years of observation of her mother's work.

Jane cited the recent national opioid crisis as an example of a unique clinical stressor that has taken a significant toll on the human and financial resources of her hospital, as many more people are seeking narcotics to self-medicate for their addictions. With greater numbers of people coming to emergency departments to receive narcotic analgesics, the young nursing leader reflected that the emergency room was rapidly becoming a site for behavioral health crises rather than for treating medical emergencies. Frequent arguments are noted between care providers and those seeking narcotics, and Jane expressed concern that these highly charged flash points may be responsible for the rise in violence that has been seen within the walls of the emergency room.

Having been in her position as a charge nurse for only three and a half years, Jane shared that she was most proud of the results seen in patient care when all members of the health-care team come together toward a common purpose to help a seriously ill patient return to better health. Her biggest challenge at her current site of employment is tied to the emotional and physical wear-and-tear that she is already experiencing, and she envisions that her clinical health-care career might last only anther five years before she explores a full-time health-care management career. With the advancing age of many providers, the decreasing joy associated with health-care delivery, and a shift toward more part-time workers, more clinicians are responding to increased workloads by preparing for nonclinical careers in health care, and some are returning to an academic environment to prepare for a professional occupation that is far removed from health-care delivery. The net effect of the many environmental challenges faced by today's clinical staff translates to quantitatively fewer providers available to care for a growing number of people requiring care, with each provider wrestling with how to find a semblance of joy from their chosen field.

Many researchers currently studying the problems associated with provider burnout and attrition point to a solution found by redefining the "treatment team," placing less pressure and reliance on traditional care providers. As retail health clinics continue to expand in number and location, and as technology continues to evolve, health-care provider roles continue to be modified. Relying on an engaged and informed health-care consumer, health-care delivery systems are allowing a great deal of self-directed care and personal management of one's own health information and sources of that information. Health literacy, where health-care consumers deepen their knowledge of how to direct care decisions in a highly complex system, is rapidly becoming a key component of health insurance companies' efforts aimed at making care consumers competent enough to help direct their own care decisions, which will result in a reduction in the total cost of care paid through health insurance premiums.[241]

Will we ever see a return to the years in which a health-care delivery career was both a vocation and an avocation? Will health-care consumers ever choose to return to the days when a health-care provider dictated a treatment plan and little else was shared with the person seeking care? In many ways, the fabric of American culture has permanently changed for the better, and those bygone days of paternalistic care are better left in the 1950s. What we should expect from today's health-care system is a coordinated effort between providers and

---

241 "Health Literacy," definition, National Network of Libraries of Medicine, accessed May 26, 2017, https://nnlm.gov/professional-development/topics/health-literacy.

consumers that focuses on the needs of the individual by designing health-care delivery solutions together. As partners in this new era of expansive technology and medical breakthroughs, the missing step remains in how the personal and very human requirements of the provider-consumer dyad will be specifically negotiated. No longer will providers feel as if the entire weight of the health-care outcome resides solely on their shoulders, and no longer should health-care consumers feel that they have been insulated from the responsibilities associated with self-care and personal self-interest. By developing a true partnership approach to the ways in which a more effective and efficient health-care experience is defined and deployed, the future care delivery team may look quite different than it does today. To assist with a smooth transition to a future state, the relationships between the many contributors will need to be clarified explicitly. As a former CEO of a large Catholic health-care system once told me, "Life's a dance, and it takes two to tango."

Key Points to Master From Chapter 13

- As health care delivery has become more complex and time pressures have become more intense, several unintended consequences have arisen, straining the social compact between health care consumers and health care providers. This new compact appears to be more transactional in nature, and begins to commoditize the health care experience.
- The impact of the new role of health care consumers in serving as activated leaders of their own treatment teams has produced unique challenges:
  - o Conflicts may arise between consumer and provider regarding diagnostic tools and therapeutic options.
  - o Consumers may rely on unscientific medical literature
  - o Mutual frustration can exist as the new relationship is defined
  - o Erosion of trust between consumer and provider may be the end result of a changing relationship.
- Providers need to embrace their roles in "principal-agent" relationships since medical information asymmetry remains a key point of misunderstanding by consumers; in a rapidly-changing and highly-complex environment, the provider needs to continue to act on the best behalf of the consumer.
- Impact to providers from the evolving trend in health care consumerism:
  - o Growing reliance on interprofessional treatment teams
  - o Erosion of trust may arise in providers just as it has in consumers
  - o Burnout is growing with a feeling of loss of provider's personal mission
  - o More advanced information technology has left some providers behind
  - o Decreased number of full time health care providers

- Providers and consumers should focus on the many strengths that have come from their unique social compact and use this bond to actively work together as aligned members of a more politically activated force for designing positive health care change.

Fourteen

WHAT LIES AHEAD?

Two Republican congressional proposals have already been kicked aside for being politically untenable to moderates who are considering the implications from the "repeal and replace" Obamacare position and its impact on their bid for reelection in the 2018 midterms. What finally passed the House with a narrow four-vote majority (217–213) was a bill that had been largely viewed as "dead on arrival" to the United States Senate, as Senator Rand Paul described it.[242] What remains to be seen is how politicians will reconcile a set of principles that will satisfy the promises made to their constituents over the past eight years balanced against the political realities that will likely result should those policy changes be implemented. The House version of the AHCA that was passed did so at the expense of significant numbers of Americans who continue to mobilize to fight against the reelection bid of any House member who supports a health-care payment reform plan that limits access, coverage, and care.

Three fundamental defects came to light in the years following the implementation of the Affordable Care Act, and these gaps in the care delivery

---

242 M. J. Lee, "Senator Rand Paul quoted in the GOP's Obamacare Replacement Bill: Dead on Arrival?," *CNN Politics*, March 8, 2017, accessed June 1, 2017, http://www.cnn.com/2017/03/07/politics/obamacare-repeal-replace-bill-congress/index.html.

system were at the heart of the "repeal Obamacare" movement that had began even prior to its approval in 2010. The first gap identified was related to health-care delivery system performance where there existed a need to improve the system's approach to fulfilling a commitment to the community to deliver high-quality care while also remaining focused on the task of creating a caring environment. Many delivery systems had already established formal quality and safety programs to identify opportunities for enhanced efficiency and effectiveness of clinical care delivery, but some systems had relegated the "softer side" of caring to an ad hoc approach that was carried mostly through the strength of a compassionate nursing staff. The expectations for patient satisfaction and loyalty were largely seen as intrinsic to the personal mission of nursing, and since nurses spent more time each day with patients and their families, it was assumed that nursing staff would provide the high-touch care necessary to supplement the more formal high-tech solutions provided by physicians.

The second gap noted following Obamacare's rollout was tied to the absence of formal connection points with community resources such as home care, retail health care, and public health supporting systems. Without these formal linkages, issues such as provision of adequate food, shelter, and home care were left to individual family members or friends to provide. As bridges began to be built between acute care providers and other less-intensive settings, objective benefits could be demonstrated such as completion of treatment plans that better realized established inpatient goals, reduction in readmissions to hospital, and enhancement of a person's overall health status.

The final gap identified by resetting a new health-care financing structure was tied to service or care gaps created because of the lack of financing for benefits not covered under ACA that were essential to a full return to an improved health status. Benefits such as medications that were needed to continue chronic care strategies, transportation to and from follow-up appointments with specialists, and availability of behavioral health services were lacking in many communities due to a lack of payment for these services. These gaps, coupled with rising health-care premiums resulting from younger and healthier individuals dropping out of insurance risk pools, gave Republicans the talking points they needed to declare that Obamacare was "a failure" and was seen to be "collapsing from its own weight" financially.

Before proceeding with potential proposals and solutions to incorporate into the health-care financing system of tomorrow, it is first important to establish a common vernacular so that these explorations can be made without the burden of disinformation created by the "Tower of Babel," in health-care parlance, that sometimes hinders our ability to move proposals forward. As the health-care debate continues on Capitol Hill, it is apparent that specific words do matter when divergent political agendas serve to separate well-intentioned elected officials from reaching a political solution that puts country before party. Some simple terms frequently bandied about but needing clarification include:

- *Health insurance:* financial resources required to pay for the health benefits needed to resolve serious illness or injury. It includes several different protections against losses from accident, medical expense, disability, or accidental death and dismemberment.[243] Typically, health insurance reflects payment of premiums to avoid ruinous costs resulting from a terrible accident or a chronic condition.[244] Misunderstandings arise when "insurance" is defined as including even routine medical care such as immunizations, minor illness treatments, routine health screening, and preventive care for which insurance was not originally intended.

- *Access to care:* one's ability to see the provider of care needed in a timely fashion and in the most appropriate clinical setting. While it is true that all Americans have access to care in some form, some sites of service, such as the nation's safety-net hospitals or community hospital emergency departments, do not provide the most appropriate level of service for comprehensive and longitudinal care solutions. As such, it is not true that all Americans can resolve their care needs equally, as insurance barriers arise when some medical offices choose

---

243 Definitions of health insurance from the Health Insurance Association of America.

244 S. M. Butler, "Why Replacing the ACA Has Republicans in a Tizzy," *Journal of the American Medical Association* 317, no. 15 (2017): 1514–1515.

not to accept certain types of health insurance. The result from this limitation in access is more costly care and more disjointed diagnostic and treatment planning. Individuals with insurance may still have difficulty with access to care should a geographically appropriate and clinically relevant provider not accept the type of health insurance coverage held by that individual. Since health-care access is typically narrowly defined by geography, providing lower-cost health insurance premiums from insurance companies located out of state may not guarantee substantial access to health-care services. Linked to this discussion is the oversimplified solution proposed by some politicians to lower the price of health insurance premiums by offering to sell the product across state lines.

*   ***Health-care services:*** the comprehensive array of appropriate diagnostic, therapeutic, and other health-promoting services that are provided in a timely fashion on behalf of a person needing those services to restore a sense of well-being and an improved health status. Coverage of specific conditions, tests, and treatments has been largely a matter of debate between Obamacare and Trumpcare solutions, since the ACA defined a set of "essential health benefits" that needed to be covered by insurance, while Republican replacement proposals have been tied to reductions in premium costs and lower out-of-pocket costs by limiting the benefits being covered.

From a political perspective, the Republican health-care agenda calls for opposition to more intrusive federal interference in private insurance markets. President Trump has largely supported many of the Republican tenets such as expansion of health savings accounts, using block grants to fund the federal portion of Medicaid programs, promoting sale of insurance across state lines, protecting those with preexisting conditions as long as individuals purchase continuous coverage, and allowing those purchasing their own insurance to deduct premium payments from their income taxes.[245] The disagreement

---

245 G. R. Wilensky, "The Future of the ACA and Health Care Policy in the United States," *Journal of the American Medical Association* 317, no. 1 (2017): 21–22.

regarding health insurance subsidies arises when debate ensues regarding the deductibility of health-care insurance premiums. Designed to help balance benefits available to private purchasers of health insurance when compared to their employer-sponsored counterparts, parity in tax benefits breaks down when one considers those making less than 250 percent of the federal poverty threshold who attempt to purchase health insurance through exchanges. In this scenario, with little tax being paid by a low-income earner, a tax deduction has much less value than it would to someone with a much higher wage. Most politicians, even those calling for repeal of the ACA, understand the need for subsidies for low-income Americans if these individuals are to continue holding health insurance, and the question that remains is how to provide the dollars to continue the subsidies. Without maintenance of some form of a tax, such as what is included in the ACA legislation, another new influx of money would have to be found to continue premium subsidies.

A separate proposal floated by some Republicans is to provide a "refundable" tax credit that would be available to Americans who pay no federal income tax, allowing many people currently being covered to maintain their health insurance coverage. In the most conservative circles, this refundable credit is viewed as a new form of entitlement, and one that should not be included in any ACA replacement plan. Without subsidies in some form, millions of people will lose insurance coverage, and the only way to fulfill President Trump's promise of limiting the number of Americans who would lose insurance coverage would be to design a plan that involves greater government-supported coverage, with payments regulated by federal sources and delivered to states as either block grants or per capita payments on behalf of these individuals.

The issue of health-care coverage as a right or a privilege continues to surface, with some opposing the term *right*, citing the strict constructionist term that applies narrowly to constitutionally assured inalienable rights that cannot be surrendered or transferred to another person, including a government.[246] Others promote health-care coverage as a right, embracing its similarity to provision of public education as a right for all Americans, helping define the

---

246 J. D. Lenchus, "The Right to Health Care," letter to the editor, *Journal of the American Medical Association* 317, no. 13 (2017): 1377.

United States as a civil society.[247] Those supporting the position of health-care coverage as a right see growing recognition over the past century of access to appropriate high-quality health-care as an essential responsibility of government on behalf of all Americans.

Despite these differences in political viewpoint, there remains an inescapable fact that some individuals carry a greater illness burden than others, and some individuals shoulder such costly expenses tied to treatment of chronic conditions that there is little hope for access to care without a well-defined strategy that provides insurance coverage using federal or state funding. It appears that two essential funding mechanisms are logical to address the needs of these individuals, and one is already in place with passage of the Affordable Care Act. The ACA spreads the financial risk of costly individuals with chronic conditions across a larger pool of insured individuals who are contributing premium payments, defining a traditional insurance model. This risk pool is funded using two primary sources that include a tax on high-income earners and the use of subsidies to assist those who cannot afford to pay the full cost of insurance premiums. The individual mandate, recently repealed as part of the Republican tax bill, helped secure payment of premiums by all individuals participating in the insurance risk pool through penalty payments placed on those who chose not to participate. A second method of providing payment for coverage is to modify the risk pools so that those with high-cost chronic conditions are managed in a separate risk pool, leaving those with lower illness burden to spread the cost of insurance coverage over a healthier and therefore less costly risk pool. The latter pool would then pay lower premium costs since they would have lower medical costs, with a result that more people might pay health insurance premiums if they were made more affordable. Those with higher-cost conditions would have their own risk pool with premium costs subsidized by a governmental agency, making their premiums more affordable. The limitation of this method is in defining how subsidies would be secured to pay for the higher-cost individuals, since the overall total cost of care would not likely be affected by simply shifting their care to a higher-risk

---

247 H. Bauchner, "Reply to a Letter to the Editor," *Journal of the American Medical Association* 317, no. 13 (2017): 1378.

pool. With fewer members covered in a high-risk pool, a new cash infusion from taxes or rationing of health-care services provided would be necessary if spending from the federal health-care budget were to remain flat.

For those supporting a reduction in the total cost of care, some have suggested that funding for new risk pools could be supported if American health-care delivery systems focused on ways in which scarce health-care resources are currently being used. Having spent $3.2 trillion on health care in the United States in 2015, accounting for 17.8 percent of the nation's gross domestic product (GDP), and with a trend that continues to escalate, consumption rates for health-care services need to be explored to look for potential savings that will offset the future growth in spending for all Americans.[248] As outlined by Emanuel, the United States is faced with undeniable health-care expenses such as paying for a growing number of older Americans with higher illness burdens, while also requiring a more strategic approach to the care of those with chronic conditions such as diabetes, cardiovascular disease, and cancer.[249] In addition, health-care spending might be downregulated if just a few additional areas of high spending could be modified, such as developing more integrated approaches to treating behavioral health conditions, providing less costly approaches to nursing home care, using public health and prevention services, and controlling the spiraling costs of pharmaceuticals.

Behavioral health conditions have long been siloed from the treatment of other medical conditions, and some states even provide legal separation of medical and behavioral health conditions by prohibiting exchange of information between mental health and traditional medical care providers.[250] Without the confluence of all health-care information into a single and integrated care plan, the treatment of behavioral health conditions is isolated from a medical framework that begs for a holistic care plan, and this defect frequently leads to

---

248 Centers for Medicare and Medicaid Services, "The National Health Expenditure Accounts (NHEA)," accessed May 1, 2017, https://www.cms.gov/Research-Statistics-Data-and-Systems/Statistics-Trends-and-Reports/NationalHealthExpendData/NationalHealthAccountsHistorical.html.

249 Emanuel, "How Can the United States Spend Its HealthCare Dollars Better?"

250 D. M. Bass, "Sharing Mental Health Records in Illinois: An Overview of Confidentiality Concerns," *Illinois Bar Association: Mental Health Matters* 1, no. 4 (2015).

errors of omission and errors of commission when drug interactions are not appreciated or when issues of medication adherence are not fully addressed. Providing comprehensive treatment plans for integrated approaches to care for these mixed medical-behavioral health conditions can significantly affect the outcome of both. Examples of such interrelated conditions include the treatment of behavioral health disorders, such as anxiety and depression, that can produce profound implications on the health outcomes seen from medical conditions such as diabetes or high blood pressure. Providers communicating a single and integrated approach to care for those with complex conditions have found opportunities that have been missed by others who have attempted to design overlapping but isolated care plans. When medical care providers have worked closely with their behavioral health compatriots to design strategies that synergistically address behavioral health conditions concomitant with chronic medical conditions, results can be seen that are more effective, efficient, and comprehensive, but such integration remains the exception rather than the rule.[251] As part of the full spectrum of solutions to approach an individual's quest for better health, consistent communication between providers regarding areas of overlap can generate better health-care outcomes at lower costs, and promote even better connections between providers and consumers of care.

Another area of opportunity to reduce expense and waste resulting from poor communication between health-care providers is the transition from an acute-care hospitalization to the long-term care facility that accepts a patient for the rehabilitative phase of an illness. Care plans are frequently incomplete and don't transition well from one site of service to the next. Failure of communication between the two sites of service is frequently manifested by a readmission to the hospital for treatment of a deteriorating clinical condition or a medical complication that arises at a nursing home site.[252,253] With anticipated

251 W. J. Katon et al., "Collaborative Care for Patients with Depression and Chronic Illnesses," *New England Journal of Medicine* 363, no. 27 (2010): 2611–2620.

252 American Health Care Association, "Hospital Readmissions," accessed May 31, 2017, https://www.ahcancal.org/quality_improvement/qualityinitiative/Pages/Hospital-Readmissions.aspx.

253 "Readmission from Skilled Nursing Facility Often Avoidable," *HealthDay*, December 22, 2016, accessed May 31, 2017, https://medicalxpress.com/news/2016-12-readmission-skilled-nursing-facility.html.

cost increases to care for an aging population, finding a way to integrate nursing home care into a comprehensive treatment plan is an essential step forward to both reduce medical expenditures and improve the level of quality provided to older and sicker Americans. One such effort aimed at making health care more strategic and efficient for these patients has been proposed through the John A. Hartford Foundation, working with the Institute for Health Improvement through a project entitled Age-Friendly Health Systems, designed to prevent harm, improve health outcomes, and lower overall costs by using evidence-based approaches to care and promoting better integration with community-based supports and services along the entire continuum of care.[254,255]

A final area of fiscal challenge that needs to be addressed by any new proposal for health-care finance reform is associated with the significant cost increases seen in prescription drugs. As the population continues to age, greater numbers of individuals with chronic medical conditions will certainly follow, and the number of prescription medications for these conditions will also increase. With both an absolute increase in the number of medications being prescribed and the advent of pharmaceutical breakthroughs in treatment of many medical conditions that are in themselves uniquely expensive, it is no accident that pharmaceutical spending has become a key area of focus for health-care finance reformers. Intravenous infusion medications and biological agents that can run into the thousands of dollars per dose are now becoming commonplace, and with an inability of the Centers for Medicare and Medicaid Services to directly negotiate price for Medicare recipients, significant increases are being seen in federal government-sponsored health-care medication costs. Pharmaceutical companies defend the prices on the grounds that the amount of money they invest to bring new breakthroughs forward is substantial and must be recovered for continued innovation to occur. The

254 John A. Hartford Foundation, "Age-Friendly Health Systems," accessed May 1, 2017, http://www.johnahartford.org/grants-strategy/current-strategies/age-friendly-hospitals/.

255 Institute for Healthcare Improvement, "Age-Friendly Health Systems: How Do We Get There?," *Health Affairs Blog*, November 3, 2016, accessed May 31, 2017, http://www.ihi.org/about/news/Pages/Age-Friendly-Health-Systems-How-Do-We-Get-There.aspx.

industry also suggests that medications have paved the way to reductions in other interventional and surgical treatments, thus reducing the total cost of care for certain conditions such as cardiovascular disease. The use of second- and third-generation pharmaceutical agents has played a significant and costly role, however, in the treatment of some medical conditions such as diabetes, where pharmaceutical expenses now account for over 60 percent of the total cost of care for this condition.[256]

One dictum still demands greater exploration when considering solutions to the rapid rise of health-care expenditures that has been seen over the past half century. Since prevention of disease and maintenance of wellness are far less costly than treatment of disease, opportunities exist to approach health maintenance as a cost-reduction strategy. Since lifestyle choices account for a significant percentage of the costs of health-care conditions that arise over the life of an individual, many have suggested that American health care should more aggressively adhere to the adage of "an ounce of prevention is worth a pound of cure."[257] Lack of exercise; obesity; high-fat and high-salt eating habits; and tobacco, alcohol, and drug abuse each represent a distinct opportunity to control cost in a more sophisticated and integrated system of care delivery. Payment for each of these self-harm behaviors appears to be vastly undervalued by policy makers, while much more costly treatments for chronic medical disorders that produce a significant financial drag on health-care budgets are seen more favorably. Investments in public health can favorably mitigate against the development of diseases tied to the risk factors listed above, and can also stave off expenses associated with treatment of very expensive medical conditions such as chronic heart disease, end-stage kidney disease, and chronic lung disease. The treatment costs for each of these long-term conditions can run into the hundreds of thousands of dollars, whereas precursor diseases such as high blood pressure and high cholesterol levels can be more successfully managed by early institution of diet, exercise, and reduction in tobacco use, each significantly less costly than treatment costs for diseases likely to result from less proactive approaches.

---

256 Emanuel, "How Can the United States Spend Its Health Care Dollars Better?"
257 B. Franklin, 1706–1790. Requoted by several, including the author's grandmother.

The risks, conditions, and expenses listed above all significantly impact the relationship between a health-care consumer and a health-care provider. In a recent Viewpoint in the *Journal of the American Medical Association,* Dr. Thomas Frieden outlined six focus areas entitled Winnable Battles that could promote greater degrees of health in a relatively brief period.[258] The six areas include approaches to conditions that could be discussed and jointly comanaged by providers and consumers and include preventable infectious diseases such as health-care-associated infections and HIV/AIDS, injuries associated with motor-vehicle accidents, chronic disease prevention associated with tobacco abuse, and teen pregnancy. In addition to these specific conditions, the United States Centers for Disease Control includes a focus area that combines nutrition, physical activity, obesity, and food safety to generally improve the overall health status of Americans. Significant reductions in the toll seen on human health have been demonstrated by creating such a focus, and these conditions should be easy enough for health professionals to implement effective strategies for, for those they serve. The main issue that continues to impede the desire of a care provider to realize the positive impact of these strategies remains a function of the unreimbursed time constraints felt by health professionals. With office visits becoming shorter due to a perceived need to see more patients at a faster pace, little allocated time is left for discussions about preventable disorders, and payment for the time needed to provide these services has not been prioritized by either private or governmental payers. This omission can be perceived by health-care consumers as reinforcement of their suspicions that providers just don't care enough to intervene, and reinforce the belief held by many providers that consumers just really don't want to participate actively in lifestyle modifications. In terms of deployment of the Winnable Battles strategies, there appears to be significant geographic variation in the use of these approaches, suggesting ongoing implementation science issues that result in an inability to capitalize

---

258 T. R. Frieden, K. Ethier, and A. Schuchat, "Improving the Health of the United States with a 'Winnable Battles' Initiative," *Journal of the American Medical Association* 317, no. 9 (2017): 903–904.

on provider-consumer relationships that focus on improvement in the health status of an entire community.

Changes in the financing of health care in this country are certainly complex, with politically charged positions accompanying a lack of specific strategies to control the overall cost of care. With a federal budget that continues to be challenged by the fiscal impact of health care, and with more Americans struggling to find the route to better health, the role of the consumer-provider dyad becomes essential in helping to better inform these evolving health-care financing discussions. As innovators design new systems to deliver higher-value health care, they will need to assure high levels of engagement of providers and consumers to have their voices heard during any discussion where changes to care systems are being proffered.

As Congress continued to mull over potential amendments to the Affordable Care Act versus a preference held by some to generate a unique solution through the American Health Care Act, one thing that was certain was that the current state was unsustainable. The plethora of possibilities to create a working health-care financing policy can be dizzying, and only the most reckless are fully confident in their predictions of the details that are likely to be seen in the future. As Einstein is quoted to have said, "When the number of factors coming into play in a phenomenological complex is too large scientific method in most cases fails. One need only think of the weather, in which case the prediction even for a few days ahead is impossible."[259] Without visionary principles to guide the future state, the dysfunctional past and murky present serve to leave the future vitality and historic success of US health care in a persistently vegetative state that will collapse under its own inefficiency. Innovative clinical scenarios that unfold every day across the country demonstrate that some care delivery systems work extremely efficiently and effectively, and some even appear to meet the Six Aims that were originally cast by the Institute of Medicine. From these successful approaches, principles can be extracted, and merging these with person-centered design principles, a more holistic approach to care delivery and its financing can be configured.

---

259 A. Einstein, German-born theoretical physicist, 1879–1955.

Before these discussions can bear fruit, however, it is important to unpack these unifying principles to develop a common framework and language that will promote focus during this vulnerable time of American health-care history. By taking an intentional approach to uncovering the "best" of health care, and by letting go of some political positions that have been carried to negotiating tables as "sacred cows," there is a high likelihood that rational people can orchestrate a health-care payment scheme that focuses on fulfilling the promise of delivering high-value health care. Not only would health-care delivery effectiveness be enhanced, but as systematic redesign recognizes the importance of consumerism and person-centered care, key requirements can be identified that will lead to even greater clinical and financial efficiency. Some of the design principles found in high-functioning health system enhancements include:

- *Promotion of a new medical neighborhood.* Much has been written about the evolving structure needed to deliver twenty-first-century health care as a "medical home" for patients where individual practitioner's offices have begun to adopt a more comprehensive approach to care delivery by incorporating a new set of provider roles that contribute to a portion of a person's care plan. When these roles are holistically combined using a systematic approach that is not limited solely to resources found in a single provider office, interdependent care teams can be created that focus on meeting the full spectrum of care needs of an individual. As these more complex teams are refined further into a true "medical neighborhood of care," simplified solutions are replaced with highly robust care planning that reaches beyond the walls of a provider's office, engaging with community resources to address both the medical needs of people and their social and environmental needs. This new set of providers spans several types of careers, and each type of provider must be recognized as an essential component of the interdependent care team, not limited in their ability to deliver care at the "top of their license." When care teams incorporate multiple respected roles into a single complex treatment team rather than encouraging providers to remain separate from one another, more robust outcomes and enriched care solutions can be realized.

- **Involved and engaged consumers of health-care services.** Not surprising, in an era of health-care consumerism, people want to play a more active role in their own health-care plan conception and execution. Using the dictum of "nothing about us without us," advocates are now demanding that better information be provided to care consumers to allow them to play a more meaningful role in developing a values-driven approach to care strategies, and in return, providers are holding those newly activated patients accountable for carrying out those care plans. From Dr. Colleen McHorney's research on medication adherence strategies, successful results have been seen in continuation of essential medications for chronic conditions when clinicians and patients focus on three key ingredients that can compose a successful medication encounter, entitled "the 3 Cs": *commitment* or *conviction* (perceived need for the medication), *concern* (addressing the perceived concern about side effects, dependency, and addiction), and *cost* (perceived affordability).[260] As health-care providers and consumers approach medication continuation using this focus on *adherence* (nonpunitive approach) to medication strategies rather than *compliance* (punitive and judgmental approach), better clinical outcomes can be seen.

- **A shift from inadequate piecemeal processes to meaningful focus on health outcomes.** At the very core of paying for the true value of health-care services is a commitment to being able to assess the results seen from each health-care encounter. For many years, health-care services have been paid for based on the number and type of care processes deployed, such as ordering a test or performing a procedure, with less regard to the final outcomes seen from such tests and

---

260 F. Smith, "Merck's Dr. Colleen McHorney's Real Life Approach to Patient Adherence Research," accessed May 2, 2017, http://www.growthconsulting.frost.com/web/images.nsf/0/FC 08DC54CE60F57986257A070053A920/$File/McKessonV3Q1fs_AdherenceInsider.html.

treatments. When care is financed based on the outcome from services delivered, the focus shifts to a care delivery experience that continues to demand favorable solutions rather than create incentives to simply deliver more services quantitatively. As part of the design of more complex health-care solutions, more favorable outcomes result when focus is paid to the economic, clinical, and humanistic (experiential) results as defined by health-care consumers. The care delivery system that can demonstrate such balanced outcomes has mastered the key tenet of delivering high-value care. This shift from simply delivering health-care services to an individual to a mind-set that embraces more comprehensive approaches toward delivery of a better health status through deployment of essential care services then produces a greater health impact for an individual and for the entire community.

- *An ounce of prevention is worth a pound of cure.* Promoting wellness and maintenance of a high degree of health requires the expenditure of fewer services to treat disease. Preventable clinical conditions that are extremely costly, such as cardiovascular disease, some forms of cancer, and metabolic syndromes such as diabetes, can take a significant toll on society. Late-stage interventions not only represent an inefficient health-care delivery system but also create a financial drag on a community. There is a significant fiscal impact from treating diseases that arise from years of poor attention to disease risk factors, and there is a significant societal toll arising from the emotional and global health burden to a community. Declines in productivity, increases in absenteeism, and a need for community programs to treat the complications arising in those with preventable illnesses can rob vital resources from a community that could be better spent in efforts to address other issues such as homelessness, hunger, and violence.

- *Becoming inclusive: the people we serve come in a variety of colors, shapes, sizes, ages, and cultures.* Using an approach of appreciative inquiry, strengths residing within a community can be recognized that will allow emerging health-care delivery networks to capitalize on people and programs that promote greater degrees of health for each community. Tomas Leon, former president and CEO of the Institute for Diversity at the American Hospital Association, has encouraged all health systems in the country to sign a pledge that reinforces that institution's commitment to community efforts toward eliminating health-care disparities. By promoting cultural competency, leadership diversity, and use of data already being collected by health systems that capture race, ethnicity, and language, some delivery systems are deploying approaches to care that better represent the multiple viewpoints of a community. The results seen from these interventions support key segments within a community that have not been traditionally heard during discussions about their community's health status. As a former health system CEO once told me, "There can be no quality without equality."[261] Like the shift seen to better recognize the needs of complex communities of color and culture are the redoubled efforts aimed at creating health systems that embrace the lives of a vibrant group of aging individuals.

Work commissioned by the John A. Hartford Foundation in New York has focused on the ways in which the care of older adults can be reimagined, thereby recognizing the unique requirements and intrinsic strengths of a growing subset of our communities. Working with the Institute for Healthcare Improvement, the Hartford Foundation has launched a pilot project that asks health systems to introduce evidence-based health practices for older citizens that promote care of higher quality and safety to favorably impact the health outcomes of seniors that will also be more cost-effective. While no results have yet been reported, this transformative approach is designed to better merge care and caring into a single, highly integrated and effective health-care experience.

- *Information systems are here to stay.* Long perceived as just repositories for the electronic storage of health information, health-care

---

261 Dr. Ram Raju, former president and CEO, New York City Health & Hospitals, personal communication, 2016.

delivery systems are now focusing on how clinical information can be used to identify care gaps, promote effective care patterns for providers, and personalize a health-care experience for individuals. "Big data" approaches have been applied to solve unique quandaries in clinical care when millions of individual episodes of care are woven together to generate databases that can be queried. From these joined data elements, clues for subsequent diagnosis and treatment plans can be recognized that had initially appeared to be only insignificant or random findings. At its most sophisticated, IBM's Watson has been commissioned to read thousands of pages of medical literature, searching for unique solutions to rare cancer conundrums, something that individual clinicians would not have ever had the time to master.[262] Using clinical decision support, information regarding the best care practices for an individual patient can be sorted to remind clinicians of the nuanced health information pertinent to an individual's health-care needs, thereby translating into practice the best approaches found from a review of medical literature as well as from the combined wisdom from thousands of previous medical encounters for similar clinical conditions.

While these design principles can be identified, it remains unclear what the ideal system for care delivery and financing in the future will look like. Social welfare debates are inherently politically charged, and changes to a health-care delivery system will likely pass through several more iterations given the complexity of the system itself and the long-standing partisanship that has evolved since Harry Truman's first experiment in proposing health-care legislation that would have provided comprehensive coverage for all Americans. At the very core of health-care financing legislation is the unassailable fact that changes to care delivery financing are wrought with probabilities to create havoc for

---

262 A. E. Cha, "Watson's Next Feat? Taking on Cancer," *Washington Post*, June 27, 2015, accessed June 5, 2017, http://www.washingtonpost.com/sf/national/2015/06/27/watsons-next-feat-taking-on-cancer/?utm_term=.ebd3a1e50ec6.

some people in our society. Those with preexisting conditions may find themselves in jeopardy should states opt out of essential care provisions or should health-care premiums for high-risk pools rise to such heights that insurance coverage, while available, becomes too expensive to purchase. If subsidies are removed, those with incomes that exceed the poverty threshold may be subject to the same fate as those with preexisting conditions, facing premiums that are more than what can be attained. Should the entire Affordable Care Act be repealed without replacement, millions of Americans will be left without health benefits that they have come to rely on as a means toward an improved health status. With all the political rancor, what appears most likely today is the addition of the following trends and supplemental changes to an evolving health-care financing system so that payment for higher-value health care can be realized. These trends are separated into those that are most likely to be implemented, those with a fair likelihood of being implemented, and those that appear to have little chance for being deployed.

The following five trends are very likely to be incorporated in near-term health financing policies:

- ***Promote insurance market competition by allowing cross-state insurance purchasing.*** This would result in a relatively minor change to the health insurance marketplace, since most health-care services delivered are through local networks of providers. Purchasing insurance benefits across state lines will promote some degree of competition between regional insurers, and this may help lower premium costs slightly. Recent proposals that call for major health insurers to consolidate suggest that health insurance will likely move in the direction of creating a few "mega" insurance plans that will be capable of providing national span through broad provider networks. Recent Federal Trade Commission rulings have stopped some of the major insurers in their efforts to consolidate, but these initial denials may be set aside should health insurers be able to demonstrate that through greater scale they can reduce the regional differences in the cost of health insurance premiums. With or without consolidation, it is unlikely to significantly impact health insurance premiums if consumers and businesses are allowed to purchase plans across traditional state lines, but it may prove to be a political win for a party in power that is desperately searching for even small health-care financing replacement victories.

- *Promote health savings accounts (HSAs).* As with selling health insurance across state lines, there is little political capital that would need to be expended to secure improvements from sponsorship of legislation regarding health savings accounts. Designed to favorably impact savings efforts, particularly of younger workers, health savings accounts will be necessary to address the increases likely to be seen in higher out-of-pocket expenses from high-deductible health plans purchased at a lower premium. The net impact of HSAs is relatively minor, since pretax dollars set aside for savings plans will be spent in consumption of health-care services at some point in the future for nearly all who choose to enroll. For HSAs to be desirable, they would need to generate a financial return that exceeds the prevailing medical inflation rate.

- *Provide financial rewards to providers who excel in all aspects of the Triple Aim (delivering high-quality care with efficiency that focuses on the consumer experience).* Exploiting the natural competitive tendencies of health systems and individual providers to distinguish themselves from their peers, rewards based on performance are a relatively uneventful addition to existing performance rewards. Provider systems have already been rewarded for "value-based purchasing" that incorporates financial gains by some providers and losses for others. The growing database on provider quality and safety and for patient experience will shed light for consumers and payers to make care decisions based on scores found for higher- and lower-performing systems. Responses from provider systems to experiments with one-sided (upside only) or two-sided (upside and downside) financial risk have been mixed, but with health-system consolidation, risk models, particularly those that limit the downside risk to providers, are logical next steps in health-care financing solutions that will focus on clinical delivery systems that hope to bear some financial risk for a greater payout.

- ***Reward innovation through funding of local and regional experiments that create multiple integrated care structures that recognize the most efficient sites of service.*** Establishing delivery structures such as medical homes and medical neighborhoods to stimulate more effective care integration appears to be an innocuous approach to health delivery system restructuring in that meaningful provider shortages appear imminent, particularly for primary-care physicians, and they could be offset by incorporating nontraditional health-care providers into the evolving care delivery networks. Defining an essential set of services will allow care integration centered on meeting the needs of relatively healthy people with high-volume, low-intensity service needs. Using retail health-care providers for such services as immunizations and treatment of common minor maladies takes the pressure off the overcrowded medical offices and allows for a shift from higher-cost sites of services (medical office practices) to lower-cost outlets (pharmacy and big-box stores). Not only does this address the emerging gap in primary-care services, it reduces the total cost of care for some health services and promotes community health solutions found in a growing "medical neighborhood" that includes more and different health-care providers.

- ***Reward health information technology solutions that promote the use of big data and personalized medicine solutions rather than reward solely for the presence of an electronic health record.*** Expanding on the promise of creating value from health information systems, and with large information-systems corporations now able to answer such a demand, out-of-the-box informatics solutions will be offered that will allow even smaller health systems and office practices to use large data sets to guide their practices and to support the delivery of high-value care with greater effectiveness and efficiency. Rewards offered through previous federal proposals have placed most providers in a position where advances in health information technology can be practically realized, leading to better communication, higher quality, and better documentation for future efforts that embrace interoperability (connectivity) of health information systems that will ultimately promote burgeoning consumerism.

The following five trends have a moderate likelihood of implementation as part of health-care finance reform:

- *Mandate continuous coverage by beneficiaries, with penalties for late enrollment.* Significant resistance was felt from many camps during the years after the implementation of the Affordable Care Act, mostly based on constitutional liberties that were felt to be affected by individual mandates. The Republican tax bill effectively removed the individual mandate and left millions of relatively healthy people to opt out from health-care coverage. When framed as penalties for late enrollment rather than as mandates for initial coverage, penalties seem quite similar to those already in place for late enrollment in Medicare for those turning sixty-five. By outlining penalties that take the form of higher premiums for a defined period should a person choose not to enroll on time, additional dollars can be generated to pay for medical expenses arising from coverage of new-onset illness as well as providing some additional funding for a national health plan and minimizing the need for significant general tax increases. Placing purchasing penalties would not replace the insurance risk pool losses that came from removal of the individual mandate, but the tactic would likely help educate young and healthy Americans about how insurance works. In addition, those without insurance who suffer from acute illnesses or injuries would provide powerful evidence to others of the value in purchasing health insurance coverage even if there were no mandate to do so.
- *Eliminate premium subsidies in favor of refundable tax credits.* Giving subsidies has always been a thorn in the side of the Republican agenda, since it is viewed as an expansion of entitlements, and use

of tax credits as an alternative support has traditionally been more palatable. The counterbalance on the side of Democrats is the view that tax credits for those with low incomes provide no real benefit, since those with lesser financial means do not typically qualify for much in the way of tax credits. The benefit of "refundable" tax credits is that they can reduce tax liabilities to less than zero, allowing for a tax refund for low-wage earners. Creating refundable tax credits also rewards those who earn a wage, even if that wage falls at near poverty levels. Making this a bit of a political football is the Republican view that even "refundable" tax credits appear to be yet another entitlement for the poor.

- *Promote public health investments that address wellness and health promotion, with a measurement system designed to validate improvements in health status.* Although public health funding might well result in lower overall costs of care, as better health and prevention strategies are associated with declines in the rates of chronic disease, there exists an issue of shortsightedness when policy makers are asked to add benefits that appear to be without specific return on investment. Most politicians have little direct knowledge about the quantitative financial benefits seen from addressing community health issues, focusing more on the addition of an incremental expense rather than the cost savings that can be seen over time when community well-being improves as part of new public health program investments are made. Another issue working against the immediate funding for public health expansion is the delay in realizing any return of investment related to public health programming, since prevention of chronic disease expense takes many years to be realized. Similarly, small-market insurers are resistant to paying for wellness programs because they are reluctant to add a perceived perquisite that might benefit a competing insurance company should the beneficiary switch to an alternate health plan. As health-care delivery teams incorporate public health strategies into an overarching approach tied to bearing clinical and financial risk, greater evidence will likely come forth that public health initiatives can yield shorter-term financial and clinical benefits, making investments in public health more palatable to politicians on both sides of the aisle.

- *Reward new models of care and caring that support an aging population.* Adoption of strategies that reduce spending for a rapidly growing segment of America makes great sense, but a large amount of political dissent already exists concerning how Medicare is viewed as an expanding entitlement program whose costs need to be reined in rather than expanded. There is no age group that is more expensive to serve than the aging senior population, but most of the rewards from funding modifications for this group will come as part of a down-regulation on excess use through the adoption of treatment guidelines based on medical evidence. Seeing this group of Americans as "superconsumers" of care, efforts will initially be aimed at reducing untoward variation in use rather than promoting new programming for seniors to consume health services differently, even if the latter strategy is more cost-effective over the long run. It is much less likely that restriction of access to services will be included in any Medicare revision given the appearance of such restrictions as "health services rationing," which will certainly bring back the discord about "death panels" that were seen during the Clinton and Obama approaches to rationalizing care.

- *Establish block grants for Medicaid funding.* As part of the second round of the American Health Care Act (AHCA, "TrumpCare," or "RyanCare"), efforts were made to promote state oversight of Medicaid through federal block grant funding with flexibility for states to define essential health-care services at a more local level. This Republican agenda item was largely viewed negatively by all Democrats and moderate Republicans as a step toward removing health-care coverage for Medicaid recipients, either by states requesting waivers to minimize their Medicaid rolls, or through efforts to more broadly define conditions that would qualify for higher premium costs when viewed as preexisting conditions. Supporters of the second iteration of the

AHCA suggested that Medicaid rolls would not be contracted since preexisting condition waivers would not likely be seen in most states, but opponents balked at supporting the bill's provision for fear that no guarantee of covering preexisting conditions could be found in the language of the bill, despite President Trump's insistence that the language was present.

Inherent in the ACA was a provision to provide start-up federal funding for up to 100 percent of program costs as part of the Medicaid expansion favored by thirty-one states. Concern for what might happen to Medicaid patients' access to providers arose when providers began dropping Medicaid patients from their practices as federal guarantees began to diminish. In 1977, when Canada shifted to block grants to support the joint federal-provincial insurance initiative that was initially launched in the 1950s, several unanticipated consequences were experienced that led to significant strains felt by provincial budgets.[263] When the federal government uncoupled its matching program to the provinces, capped the annual growth rate for payments, and provided for one-time reductions in federal block grant support in 1982, the provinces felt considerable budgetary constraints that complicated an economy that was already experiencing sluggish growth. In the United States, with a Medicaid program that enjoys richer benefits than the program in place in Canada, the impact from alteration in federal funding contributions would produce even more of a fiscal strain on state budgets. In addition, despite Speaker Ryan's insistence that block grants would allow for greater flexibility and proper incentives that reinforce improvements in service delivery, the experience in Canada suggests that when financial stresses arose, the provincial governments reduced payments to hospitals and renegotiated physician pricing through intense bargaining. In the United States, as has already been seen in some regions, when Medicaid

---

263 B. D. Sommers, "Medicaid Block Grants and Federalism: Lessons from Canada," *Journal of the American Medical Association* 317, no. 16 (2017): 1619–1620.

reimbursement is perceived as insufficient, American providers simply close their practices to Medicaid patients, thereby creating significant issues for those already suffering from poor access to care.

The following five tactics are much less likely to be implemented given the current political climate:

- *Establish high-risk pools that promote disease management and cost efficiency, and eliminate the ACA's preexisting exclusion regulations.* This approach had been included in the House version of the AHCA, establishing high-risk pools at a state level that were designed to allow healthier individuals to purchase health care through state-based insurance exchanges at lower premium costs than found in the ACA.[264] While this approach appears to make sense, removing high-cost patients from the larger risk pool and establishing a separate high-risk pool is somewhat shortsighted when facing the growing subsidies needed to care for such an expanding pool of patients. There is no evidence that the illness burden of America is lessening, and in fact, much has been written about the explosion of health-care expenditures that are to be expected due to an aging population, coupled with several emerging conditions such as childhood obesity and behavioral health disorders that will result in greater numbers afflicted with chronic illnesses and medical expenses. Estimates currently are that 5 percent of patients under sixty-five years of age account for nearly 50 percent of all expenditures for that age group,[265] leading to a need for a substantial initial infusion of state funding to secure appropriate coverage for such high-risk pools. Such pools with high illness burden

---

264 R. E. Herzlinger, B. D. Richman, and R. J. Boxer, "Achieving Universal Coverage without Turning to a Single Payer: Lessons from 3 Other Countries," *Journal of the American Medical Association* 317, no. 14 (2017): 1409–1410.

265 E. M. Mitchell, "Concentration of Health Expenditures in the US Civilian Noninstitutionalized Population, 2014," Agency for Healthcare Research and Quality, Statistical Brief #497, accessed May 2, 2017, https://meps.ahrq.gov/data_files/publications/st497/stat497.shtml.

have been used by states for nearly four decades, covering approximately one hundred thousand individuals at a cost of over \$1 billion annually.[266] Compared to the plan offered by the Republicans in the House who were proposing significantly less funding on a per capita basis, the historic financing data used in previous experiments applies to a more selected group of individuals where highly restrictive qualification standards were established to minimize the number of people eligible for high-risk pool coverage. The impact from such restrictions made it likely that the House proposal significantly underestimated the overall financial impact from creating high-risk pools.

Regarding preexisting conditions, there does appear to be some enthusiasm from the Republicans for removing the preexisting condition exclusions found in the 2010 ACA legislation. Initially seen as a deal breaker by both political parties, traction to remove the language barring community ratings for those with preexisting conditions seem to be offset by an amendment to the AHCA that allows for the establishment of a special \$8 billion infusion over five years to cover those individuals who stood to lose benefits. The modified AHCA allowed states to seek a waiver that would allow insurers to return to previous underwriting practices that focused on denial of coverage to an individual with a preexisting condition. Since most people with preexisting conditions are insured through employer-based plans, Republicans suggest that the actual number of people affected by removing the rollback against preexisting conditions would be quite small, when in fact the number of Americans who may be compromised without access to insurance is in the millions. The Kaiser Family Foundation estimated that actions taken by insurers to exclude those with preexisting conditions using underwriting criteria would affect a minimum of 8 percent of the nonelderly population, with many more being affected

---

266 Henry J. Kaiser Family Foundation, "Health Reform: High-Risk Pools for Uninsurable Individuals," February 22, 2017, accessed May 4, 2017, http://kff.org/health-reform/issue-brief/high-risk-pools-for-uninsurable-individuals/.

should job loss occur.[267] Since fifty-two million Americans suffer from some form of preexisting condition, the overall pool of vulnerable people who may develop a condition that renders them uninsurable is much higher than proposed by the Republican legislation. This group has the potential of losing employer-based coverage because of job loss, and it includes young adults turning twenty-six years of age and those losing coverage because of divorce. Superimposed on this pool are those who are uninsured given their employment by firms that do not offer group health insurance coverage. Those who are self-employed or retiring before becoming eligible for Medicare would also be affected.

Since the ACA solved the underwriting predicament of 18 percent of Americans who were excluded from insurance and sought health coverage in the individual markets before 2010, removing the language that rolls back preexisting condition limitations affects a very large portion of the country. Since denials based on health conditions, specific medications, and risky occupations are quite prevalent, it is not just the unique condition that leads to a nonqualification status for medical insurance. Even if those with a preexisting condition were to be offered some minimal coverage, insurance companies frequently write in special riders that allow them to exclude portions of traditional benefits for individuals. Strategies used by companies to reduce richness of benefits include tactics such as excluding coverage for the body parts affected by the preexisting condition, hiking rates for premiums, raising deductible thresholds to much higher levels, or limiting coverage of certain prescription drugs. Even relatively uncomplicated conditions have fallen under the preexisting condition language, leaving potential applicants unable to secure medical insurance. One such example was cited in research carried out by the

267 Henry J. Kaiser Family Foundation, "Health Reform: Pre-existing Conditions and Medical Underwriting in the Individual Insurance Market Prior to the ACA," December 12, 2016, accessed May 4, 2017, http://kff.org/health-reform/issue-brief/pre-existing-conditions-and-medical-underwriting-in-the-individual-insurance-market-prior-to-the-aca/.

Kaiser Family Foundation when they submitted a medical insurance application to several medical insurers on behalf of a hypothetical person with seasonal allergies, an extremely common and mild medical condition that frequently requires no medical intervention with the exception of periodic over-the-counter oral medications.[268] Of the sixty applications submitted, only three were offered standard coverage, five were fully declined, and the remainder were offered exclusion riders that limited coverage for upper respiratory tract conditions of any type. A subgroup was offered coverage but with premium rates that were 25 percent higher than standard pricing.

- *Cap the tax benefit on employer-based health plans.* So-called "Cadillac" health plans with very rich benefits were taxed as part of the ACA. The proposed AHCA plan, calling for limitations on the deductibility of employer-sponsored health insurance premiums being paid by business, was projected to be a more progressive form of the Cadillac tax since it passed the tax along to employees based on their income. Some American voters have expressed concern about paying for expanded health-care coverage, either through global federal budgets or through state-based high-risk pools, with a belief that the plan provides an entitlement benefit for the jobless that comes directly from the paychecks of those who are working.

- *Create an independent health board to define essential health services and to define and reward the best evidence-based practices.* An idea floated by then-senator Tom Daschle from South Dakota in 2008, an independent national health board would be convened to identify essential health benefits while also promoting incentive payments for the use of widely accepted and evidence-based care patterns.[269] This body, operating much like the Federal Reserve Board, which oversees

---

268 Henry J. Kaiser Family Foundation, "Health Costs: How Accessible Is Individual Health Insurance for Consumer in Less-Than-Perfect Health?," June 1, 2001, accessed May 4, 2017, http://kff.org/health-costs/report/how-accessible-is-individual-health-insurance-for-2/.

269 T. Daschle, S. S. Greenberger, and J. M. Lambrew, *Critical: What We Can Do about the Health-Care Crisis* (New York: Thomas Dunne Books).

highly complicated financial matters, would be insulated from political pressure, yet it would still be accountable to elected officials and
the American people. Creating a single standard of care to be delivered
to every person in the country, there would be a defined set of services
that would be mandated for payment by public and private payers.
Like the body that advised the state of Oregon when it experimented
with services designated to be of highest value for the state's Medicaid
program, the national health advisory board would comprise a variety of health professionals and business representatives who would be
the final arbiter of benefits covered based on the relative value and
impact of health-care services. Speaking against such a proposal are
small-government conservatives who favor a free-market solution with
less governmental interference, since a national health board would be
the antithesis of free-market forces. Although such a council has not
been incorporated into either the Affordable Care Act or the American
Health Care Act, its impact may be felt should a single-payer solution
come forward or if federal oversight of state-based programs is needed
if and when block grants are used for funding Medicaid.

- *Negotiate pharmaceutical costs at scale.* Perhaps no other body
has negotiated harder and more effectively on Capitol Hill than the
pharmaceutical lobbyists, who have been able to successfully keep
medication coverage provisions generally intact. As part of the original proposal for Medicare and during federal health plan proposals
during the Clinton and Obama White Houses, representatives of the
pharmaceutical industry successfully persuaded Congress to exclude
any provision that would allow direct negotiation of pharmaceutical
prices by federal health programs, mainly under the aegis that the
government has an inherent conflict when it represents itself in negotiating drug prices in a free-market economy. Citing that reductions
in drug prices would lead to reductions in pharmaceutical innovation, the drug companies have successfully lobbied to have government keep its distance from big pharma firms with respect to pricing
parameters contained in federal programs. Estimates suggest that

between \$16 and \$20 billion each year could be squeezed out of government health programs if drug prices were to be made eligible for negotiation in programs such as Part D Medicare, which pays as much as 80 percent more for medications than medications purchased using the Department of Veteran Affairs benefits.[270,271]

- ***Reward care systems that demonstrate an ability to promote health literacy while implementing approaches to care that recognize cultural diversity.*** Reducing unwarranted variation in use by rewarding consumers for more effectively using the American health-care system seems like an outstanding idea, but little data are currently available demonstrating the financial benefit of doing so. It seems intuitively brilliant to better understand unique characteristics of a system that could be improved if services were more sensitively delivered to a more highly medically literate population. The primary barrier to such a program is the costs incurred to train local educators how to teach segments of their communities about the better use of the health-care services available to them. Small pilot programs have demonstrated some success in decreasing unwarranted variation, such as the Latino diabetes initiative in South Bend, Indiana, where costs associated with use of emergency department services for primary-care complaints associated with diabetes mellitus decreased significantly. In response to changing sites of service for this chronic condition, reductions in uncompensated care were also seen, attributed to a program for uninsured immigrants that improved both clinical care and satisfaction with care services.[272] Seen as an incremental expense for an already costly set of covered services, federal assistance is not likely, and similar

270 Editorial Board, "Let Medicare Negotiate Drug Prices: Our View," *USA Today*, April 20, 2014, accessed June 1, 2017, https://www.usatoday.com/story/opinion/2014/04/20/medicare-part-d-prescription-drug-prices-negotiate-editorials-debates/7943745/.

271 E. Pianin, "Medicare Could Save Nearly \$26 Billion a Year Negotiating Drug Prices," *Fiscal Times*, March 9, 2017, accessed June 1, 2017, https://finance.yahoo.com/news/medicare-could-save-nearly-16-221300487.html.

272 L. Batani, M. DeMont, and K. Anderson, *The Latino Diabetes Initiative. Impact on Economic, Clinical, and Humanistic Metrics Using a New Model of Care* (Memorial Health System, 2006).

to public health programming designed to improve the overall health of a community, new programs such as these are more likely to be paid through private foundation grants or as pilot projects using small amounts of federal funding made available through the Center for Medicare and Medicaid Innovation (CMMI).

Getting the new health system design correct is important to the millions of people who rely on delivery of high-quality services every day to sustain and improve human life. Being able to discern the best care delivery system is part and parcel of America's position in the world as an exemplar of innovation, entrepreneurship, and leadership. Much like the image that our country projects to the world demonstrating what is possible in governance, business, human rights, and scientific discovery, American health care has long been emulated as the best systematic approach to treatment of health conditions found in the history of the world's civilizations. The inflection point at which this country finds itself can be viewed through the lens of an optimist from which our scientific prowess, information technology, creativity, and advances in all fields from birth to death are unparalleled.

However, our current position can also be viewed somewhat less optimistically as a reflection of a key moment in history when American health care became available only to the privileged few, based on income, protected class, or employment status. One must wonder if the very fabric of America will be tested, just as with the many great revolutions found in other great societies that were challenged in the past, when growing disparity in America between those privileged enough to enjoy the highly valued benefits from outstanding health-care services will be separated from a growing number of individuals who find that an improved health status lies just beyond their reach. Early signs point to the latter as rising rates of homelessness, joblessness, hunger, and gun violence all serve as early signals of one of the most disturbing indicators of all, that the life-span of an American has begun to shorten despite the impressive technological advances that have been promoted.[273] Not only are

273 D. Squires, "The Shortening American Lifespan," *To the Point: Quick Takes on Health Care Policy and Practice,* The Commonwealth Fund, January 4, 2017, accessed April 28, 2017.

these changes in life expectancy noteworthy and disturbing, but the distribution within the country's microenvironments of cities and states suggests that income-based disparities in life expectancy are large and growing rapidly. The most important set of digits that are associated with length of life are not tied to blood pressure or diabetes control, but rather to the zip code into which you are born. What had been a shared expectation of a longer length of life that would approach one hundred years for most Americans has now reversed, largely from changes in health status associated with obesity, rates of diabetes, the impact from an array of environmental factors, and inequities in availability of essential health-care service.[274]

Caught in the middle of the health-care debate are the health-care provider and health-care consumer, struggling to continue a relationship that has generated miraculous results for hundreds of years. Essential to the current health-care debate are the voices of those most affected by the changes that are needed to allow our great country to continue to fund health care for as many Americans as possible. Without a thoughtful approach to payment redesign, this country may find itself falling victim to an unsustainable economic and social challenge that produces a health-care revolution to answer with finality the question of whether high-value health care is a right for all Americans or whether it is a privilege for a just a few to enjoy. Perfecting a system for health-care financing is one of the most critical challenges facing politicians today, not just to address the emerging crises seen from an imbalanced federal budget, but for the very survival of all Americans engaged in the dance of life, where consumers and providers of care remain the most intimate of partners.

---

274 S. J. Olshansky et al., "A Potential Decline in Life Expectancy in the United States in the 21st Century," *New England Journal of Medicine* 305, no. 11 (2005): 1138–1145.

Key Points to Master from Chapter 14

- The Affordable Care Act (ACA) had three key gaps:
    - Health care delivery system quality performance was not intimately tied to the creation of an environment for caring.
    - Formal connection points between acute health care delivery environments and the community were not assured.
    - Key benefits that promoted a return to an improved health status were not included in the ACA, such as coverage for medications, transportation, and assuring access to key medical services.
- Three key definitions needed to understand before discussing the future state solutions in health care financing:
    - Health Insurance: The financial resources required to pay for the health benefits needed to resolve serious illness or injury.
    - Access to care: One's ability to see the provider of care in a timely fashion and in the most appropriate clinical setting.
    - Health care services: The comprehensive array of appropriate diagnostic, therapeutic, and other health-promoting services provided in a timely fashion to restore well-being.
- Solutions that do not call for integration of medical and behavioral health services are less likely to provide for meaningful, effective, and efficient care plans to be successfully executed.
- Several key components are needed to coordinate care along the continuum between acute care hospitals and post-acute care settings:
    - Promotion of outstanding communication channels.
    - Joint improvement activities between acute and subacute care facilities is an essential component of fully integrated care
    - Efforts to utilize a common information technology platform are associated with more effective and efficient information exchange.
- Prescription costs are rapidly rising and contribute mightily to the overall total cost of health care services.
- Preventive services can be cost-effective to include as plan benefits if they include approaches to common lifestyle conditions such as diet, exercise, and self-harm habits such as tobacco, drug, and alcohol abuse.

- "Winnable Battles" promote greater degrees of health in a relatively brief time:
  - Preventable infectious diseases: health care-associated infections, HIV/AIDS
  - Injuries from motor vehicle accidents
  - Chronic disease prevention associated with tobacco use
  - Teen pregnancy
  - Nutrition, physical activity, obesity, and food safety
- Design principles for high-functioning health systems:
  - Promotion of a new medical neighborhood
  - Those we serve need to be involved in the design of health systems
  - Health outcomes should be the focus rather than just care processes
  - An ounce of prevention is worth a pound of cure
  - Become more inclusive of the many people being served in the community
  - Information systems are here to stay
- Five trends most likely to be seen in near-term health financing policy:
  - Purchasing health insurance across state lines
  - Health Savings Accounts
  - Financial rewards for those systems who excel in all aspects of the Triple Aim
  - Rewards for local and regional experiments to test integrated care structures that reinforce the most efficient care sites of service
  - Reward health information technology that promotes the use of Big Data to personalize solutions with higher degrees of effectiveness and efficiency
- Five trends with moderate likelihood of adoption in legislation include:
  - Mandating continuous coverage for beneficiaries; penalties for late enrollment
  - Eliminate premium subsidies in favor of refundable tax credits
  - Promote health and wellness with a measurement system to assess impact
  - Reward new models of care that better support an aging population

- o   Establish block grants for Medicaid funding
- Five trends less likely to be adopted in near term legislation:
  - o   High-risk pools and elimination of pre-existing condition exclusions
  - o   Capping the tax benefit for employer-based health plans
  - o   Creation of an independent board to oversee essential health services
  - o   Negotiating pharmaceutical costs in all federal health plans
  - o   Rewarding health systems that focus on health literacy and diversity

Epilogue

In Paul Starr's recent publication *Remedy and Reaction*, he notes that the United States has a long history of leaving large populations without health insurance coverage, and the number of Americans who are without health-care coverage neared fifty million by 2010.[275] This large gap in coverage, accompanied by greater consumption of the gross domestic product needed to pay for health-care spending, has worsened over the past thirty years, leaving policy makers unable to design a system for payment that provides essential services for most Americans without producing an untenable impact on the federal budget. As new proposals have been presented, ideological warfare has erupted that has involved a variety of interested parties to create a workable system to pay for the spiraling costs of health care. Starr cites an evolving *policy trap* of an increasingly costly and complicated system where entrenched representatives from many health-care sectors create complexity that makes it difficult to change the care delivery experience.

The vitriol that has sprung forward since the Obamacare plan came to life in 2010 percolated below the surface until the 2016 election, when Donald Trump and a Republican congressional majority were elected to office. Stories of political hostility at the time when the Affordable Care Act was proposed have been replaced with derisive language that includes "alternative facts" and highly partisan actions. New mobs of angry citizens now crowd congressional town hall meetings demanding that Obamacare be preserved. This shift in the populist opinions concerning the 2010 health-care bill largely stems from a poor understanding that Obamacare and the Affordable Care Act are synonymous, with some people calling specifically for Obamacare to be repealed and replaced while also encouraging maintenance of the Affordable Care Act. Even Republican members of Congress have now come to the defense of key provisions of the ACA, especially those portions excluded in the proposed Republican health-care financing bill calling for restrictions on limitations of

---

275 P. Starr, *Remedy and Reaction: The Peculiar American Struggle Over Health Care Reform*, revised edition (New Haven, CT: Yale University Press, 2013).

preexisting conditions. Another point of agreement for most Republicans was in preservation of the Obamacare provision allowing younger adults to remain on their parents' insurance policy until age twenty-six. For many politicians on both sides of the aisle, the ugly truth that nearly twenty million people could lose health-care coverage if the ACA were repealed created significant political risk. Democrats have been taking the lead to remind the electorate that should the ACA be repealed without an adequate replacement, those same people who would lose insurance coverage would be very motivated to come out to vote during midterm elections to voice their objections to losing their coverage.

Amid all this political football, the question that remains on the minds of average Americans is related to the personal consequences from any proposal that terminates or significantly limits coverage for some segments of American society. For those losing coverage, the main question centers on their personal financial security and what financial protections will exist in whatever health-care reform bill may come next. Over the past thirty years, several experiments have been tried to design systems to modify the payment schemes for health-care services. The result of these efforts has been to create an unsustainable financial system that further promotes spiraling health-care costs. The lines in this battle have been passionately drawn, leading to today's health-care system, which is both ineffective and inefficient when compared to other industrialized nations, and it leaves millions of Americans at risk of medical bankruptcy should a catastrophic or chronic illness befall their family. What has been missing from the debate about health-care policy has been a frank discussion of how new payment systems affect the very people directly involved on both ends of the stethoscope. Care providers have changed their delivery practices in response to health-care financing policies, and those receiving care have lamented the significant changes to the long-standing social compact with their providers, leaving all parties disillusioned and confused.

As partisan politics continue to provide fireworks on Capitol Hill during debates on health-care funding, there are noteworthy disagreements about how best to cover the cost of expensive but essential medical services. Policy decisions are being made that affect the types and numbers of services that will be covered, who can provide those services, how care can be subsidized for those who cannot afford essential services, and even how to balance expanded coverage against cost controls. Not all funding proposals will survive congressional debate, and the impact from changes to health-care delivery systems will not be solely limited to how these systems are financed. The greater concern for providers and consumers of care is related to the many ways that these policies change the primacy of the care experience itself, with a great divide now being created between providers and consumers that has eroded the intrinsic bond between the two groups. When interviewed, both providers and consumers express regret about the ways in which the funding of health care has interfered with one of the most intimate of all transactional relationships, and they express dissatisfaction with the direction of their unique and delicate relationship.

Preservation of the provider-consumer compact is a core element of how American health care can return to its position of prominence and respect on the world stage. By focusing more on the care experience rather than viewing it solely as a business transaction, we can achieve better health outcomes when the two parties unite in pursuit of finding the "best" answer to a personal health conundrum. Policy makers, funders, and suppliers need to rely on providers and consumers to join them in working through solutions to the health-care financing crisis that can better establish the true value of a health-care experience. Borrowing from an adage in health-care process design, consumers and their providers are expressing strong desires that "nothing about us should be done without us." By casting the health-care experience first as a relationship between two parties who are intimately joined in the pursuit of better health, we can reestablish the bond between care participants with more satisfying results. With this social compact assured, engaged providers and consumers can assist in redesigning care experiences that meet the goals established by the Institute of Medicine when that group first defined high-quality health care.

"Care with caring" remains alive and well in the hearts of most health-care providers, and the emotional bond with health-care consumers is essential as the country attempts to answer the larger challenge of how to provide comprehensive health care for most Americans. At critical times like these, I return to the sage wisdom of my old mentor, Dr. Jeremy Swan, who challenged me to never forget how to use the most important instrument that I possess when examining a patient's heart: my own heart.

Acknowledgments

I decided to memorialize a lifetime of working in many diverse corners of health care so that you, the reader, might better engage in the meaningful dialogue that is required to create a more comprehensive approach to care delivery that will allow each of us to benefit from all that American health care has to offer. I want to thank the reader in advance for your interest in helping to create a health care system that has heart and retains the best of its human qualities. I challenge each of you to jointly participate actively as those who deliver care and those who receive it, so that your voices will be heard. Through these discussions, all of us will benefit from the best that America health care has to offer; by joining in the debate regarding health care system redesign, you can help to ensure that the heart of health care will be retained.

I want to thank my wife, Dyan, and my children for providing their love and ongoing support for this project, and for the countless hours of reading and comment that helped bring the final perspectives I needed to bring this book to life.

I had many mentor-friends who stimulated my thinking at every turn of my career, and you each have my heartfelt appreciation and undying support for all that you did to make me want to explore my thinking more deeply. I give special recognition to my undergraduate advisor, Dr. James VanAllen, who suggested that I was more suited for applied life sciences than the physics career path on which I originally embarked, and for the authors and artists of the University of Iowa Writers Workshop, especially June Melby, who taught me to dream and to commit those dreams to paper. To Dr. James Shehan who taught me to take the pursuit of medicine seriously, providing me the challenge I needed when he suggested that I would never become a physician, but later rewarding me by referring his patients to my specialty practice. To Jeff Peterson and Mark Nadaud who organized a medical school study group to help smooth the road as we attempted to master the educational requirements we needed during our careers.

Further thanks are given to Drs. Bruno Masters and John Nansen and all of my fellow residents during my initial transition to health care delivery, but especially to Dr. Bill Ankeny and Dr. Larry Baker who helped provide laughter during the 115 hour work weeks of internship. To my internal medicine residency comrade, Dr. Bob Beveridge, a special thanks for your kind words, your great laughter, and the sharing of an occasional Canadian brew. To all of the fellows, staff, residents, and students with whom I interacted during my formal training, but especially Drs. Shaul Massry, Lakhi Sakhrani, and Nachman Brautbar, my mentors who personally encouraged a deep exploration of the field of nephrology so that I felt prepared for clinical practice.

There were many who helped me prepare for my second career in health care administration, including Drs. David Kindig and Fitzhugh Millan, who helped me appreciate the history and politics of health care, while also challenging me to build a more comprehensive and inclusive system of caring. A special thanks to Drs. Preston Strosnider, Chris Yetter, David Masuda, and Steve Brazeel, also known as the Back Row Bums at the University of Wisconsin, for providing comedic relief and innovative thinking during the two year intensive that culminated in a masters degree in medical administration. In my administrative medicine career, I had the opportunity to interact with many exceptional and high-performing individuals, but I would be remiss if I didn't offer a special thank you to Bruce Greenberg who taught me about health care payment systems in his role as CEO of a provider-owned health plan, and to Phil Newbold, Reg Wagle, Diane Stover, and Mike O'Neil who stretched my thinking regarding health care experience design through their work in the Innovation Café of Memorial Health System. I would also like to thank my colleagues at NorthShore University HealthSystem for giving me an opportunity to help improve the quality and safety systems that were already operating at a high level. While there, Dr. Ned Wagner, Tony Solomonides, and Tom Smith provided valuable editorial review that stimulated many revisions to this manuscript, and Mike Raymond, Ray Grady, Jesse Peterson-Hall, Maureen Kharasch, Liz Behrens, Jeff Vender, Mark Talamonti, John Howington, and Bernard Ewigman who also contributed to my understanding of health care quality. To my associates at the American Hospital Association, especially Maulik Joshi, Heather Jorna, Neil Jesuele, and Rich Umbdenstock who provided guidance and enthusiasm for my interest in public health and research. While there, I had the great fortune of learning from the masterful wisdom of a true gentleman scholar, Dr. Larry Prybil, who reminded me of those we have been called to serve, and how success is best realized when professional divides are spanned through multilateral collaboration. A special thanks also goes to Paul Starr and Don Berwick for challenging me with their viewpoints documented from years of academic research.

Most importantly, I would like to thank my patients and their families, who reminded me daily of the importance of maintaining the delicate human elegance that is so essential to creating magnificent health care experiences.

About the Author

Kenneth P. Anderson, DO, MS, CPE is an author and educator who practiced clinical nephrology and transplant medicine, with nearly thirty five years of health care experience. A graduate of the University of Iowa, he was initially on a path to a career in physics, but realized the impact that applied life science had on his personal mission to help those in need of health care who had difficulty with access to and the cost of health care. After graduating from the College of Osteopathic Medicine and Surgery, now known as Des Moines University, Anderson completed a three year family medicine residency at the University of Iowa's Lutheran Hospital campus where he also served as chief resident. Having developed strong research and clinical interest in nephrology, he enrolled at Yale University's Norwalk Hospital where he completed an internal medicine residency program where he also served as chief resident. He completed his formal training in nephrology at the University of Southern California-Los Angeles County Hospital, moving to Des Moines, Iowa to serve as managing partner of a private practice in acute and chronic kidney care while serving as transplant nephrologist for the kidney and heart transplant programs at Mercy Hospital Health System.

While in clinical practice, Anderson served on the Iowa State Board of Health, chaired the Network XII Quality Committee for a four-state region of the Health Care Finance Administration, and advised Senator Tom Harkin and the Clinton Administration on matters regarding health care reform. He served as section chief for nephrology and assistant department chairman for internal medicine, served as a member of two hospital boards, and became chief of the medical staff. While serving in this capacity, he completed a certificate program through Harvard University and received his masters degree in administrative medicine from the University of Wisconsin.

Anderson's formal administrative career began in South Bend, Indiana, where he served as chief medical officer for PARTNERS National Health Plans of Indiana and as vice president for quality and safety at Memorial Health System. During this time, he became a senior examiner for the Baldrige Performance Excellence Program, serving on a number of national

269

and regional quality and safety organizations including the Indiana Patient Safety Council.

As chief medical quality officer at NorthShore University HealthSystem in Chicago's northern suburbs, Dr. Anderson provided oversight to quality and safety activities for the two-thousand, five-hundred physician member medical staff of a four hospital health system, started a quality fellowship program designed to train future medical staff leaders, and co-directed the Center for Clinical Research Informatics. Recruited as chief operating officer and interim chief executive officer for the American Hospital Association's Health Research and Education Trust, he served as principal investigator for a number of national research contracts from the Centers for Medicare and Medicaid Services and the Center for Medicare and Medicaid Innovation.

Anderson retired from his administrative positions in 2017, and now lives in Iowa City, Iowa, with his wife, Dyan, and their dog Bette. Anderson continues to write, teach, and stimulate others to design health care systems with heart.